The Busy Woman's
21-Day Guide
to Clean Eating

The Busy Woman's
21-Day Guide
to Clean Eating

DR. JAMIE HARDY

The Lifestyle Pharmacist ™

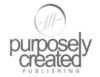

purposely
created
PUBLISHING

THE BUSY WOMAN'S 21-DAY GUIDE TO CLEAN EATING

Published by Purposely Created Publishing Group™

This content of this book is for informational and educational purposes only. Please consult with your physician for official medical advice.

The recipes in this guide are inspired by and adapted from some of my favorite cookbooks, cooking shows, and magazines. Of course, I put a special twist on them to make them clean and lean.

Printed in the United States of America

ISBN: 978-1-945558-59-7

Special discounts are available on bulk quantity purchases by book clubs, associations, and special interest groups. For details email: sales@publishyourgift.com or call (888) 949-6228.

For information logon to: www.PublishYourGift.com

Dedication

This book is dedicated to my 98-year-old granny, who has been patiently waiting for me to tell her that I am having a baby. So with the completion of this project, I can honestly say that I have given birth to a baby of sorts—my first published book. This labor of love would not have been possible without the inspiration and prayers of my granny, encouragement from my husband, and unwavering support from my mom, dad, sister, and auntie. The arrival of this "baby" is because of all of you!

What you eat, drink, and how you treat your body affects your health and ultimately the quality of life you live. My mission is to teach busy young women how to eat healthier, effectively manage stress, and incorporate exercise into their lifestyle so they can be fit, fabulous, and fulfilled without prescribed pills.

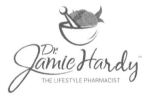

Table of Contents

Table of Contents

Who This Book Is For

The Busy Woman's 21-Day Guide to Clean Eating is for the busy entrepreneur, leader, professional, mom, wife, fiancé, and girlfriend who is hard at work being everything to everyone EXCEPT for YOURSELF. You often put your needs on hold to take care of others. The constant pressures at work, the never-ending to-do lists, and the stress of trying to juggle it all are taking a toll on you.

Do you seek refuge from your pain and disappointment in a gallon of homemade vanilla ice cream, a dozen glazed doughnuts, or a bucket of crispy fried chicken? Do you toss and turn at night, unable to clear your mind, and wake up exhausted every morning? Are caramel macchiatos, sodas, and afternoon energy drinks the only way you can make it through the day? Are you feeling guilty about the sweet, salty, and fat-filled foods that you eat on a daily basis? Are you frustrated and overwhelmed at the thought of giving your lifestyle a much-needed makeover?

If any of that rings a bell, then this book is for YOU!

Introduction

I've been there too—busy juggling a career, a business, and a relationship. Escaping trauma and despair in unhealthy ways. Trying to heal myself in unhealthy ways. In this book, I reveal the strategies that I used to take back my health and my life. I practice what I teach, so trust and believe that I'm not telling you to do anything that I don't do in my everyday life.

In this guidebook, I offer help and hope for breaking the cycle of unhealthy eating that so many women face every day. Right now, there is a woman telling herself that her jam-packed schedule leaves no time for eating clean. She has convinced herself that there is no way she can look for healthy recipes, then shop for the ingredients, and *then* cook. She is 100 percent certain that it is impossible to fit any of that into her schedule. She believes that eating from the drive-thru, frozen food section, and restaurant take out is best for her lifestyle because that saves her time. What's the harm in that?

Researchers and healthcare providers agree that many of the illnesses and chronic diseases plaguing our bodies are preventable. There is scientific evidence linking the trans and saturated fat in foods to heart disease and stroke. The connection between obesity and diabetes is well established. The alarmingly high amount of salt that is consumed on a daily basis is without question related to the high blood pressure so many people are diagnosed with.

It is time for women to clean up their act and take ownership of the long-term health effects of dirty eating habits. I realize that taking the clean eating leap can be scary and overwhelming. No worries. I am right here with you along this journey to give you tips, tricks, and a few shortcuts along the way. You have taken the biggest step already. You purchased this book, which signals that you are open to making a change. That is hurdle #1, and you have already jumped over it!

So here is what you can expect from me. I will break down the meaning of clean eating in a way that is practical and easy to understand. I will hand you a mirror that allows you to take a closer look at the way you are treating your body through the foods that you eat. Most importantly, I will provide a solution for transforming the way you eat, one meal at a time, for 21 days. *The Busy Woman's 21-Day Guide to Clean Eating* is designed to tell you what to eat, when to eat, and how to cook it. I am finally living the life of my dreams, and so can you! Let's get started.

Smooches,

Dr. Jamie

....

The Busy Woman's
21-Day Guide to Clean Eating
PART 1

....

The Dream Became a Nightmare

Armed with a Prescription and a Plan

An Alternative Strategy

The Dream Became a Nightmare

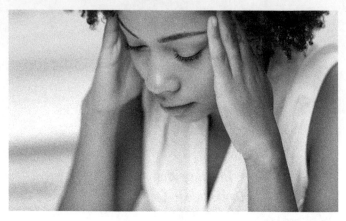

I was in my mid-20s and living what most people would call a dream life. I was a doctor with a successful career. I was living in a newly built home. I was driving a luxury car. I had been on numerous international vacations. I was dating the man of my dreams. I had it all...or so I thought. There was just one problem: me in the mirror. I barely recognized the reflection staring back at me. Who was *this* woman? She can't be *me*. I'm perfect. I have it all together. WRONG. The truth is that my life was in shambles. I couldn't eat, sleep, or even think. I was angry, humiliated, and so incredibly sad. I was tired of crying, tired of hurting, and tired of living with the pain. I was embarrassed that this was happening to me. How could this be happening to me? I wanted to end it all.

The reality is that I was in a deep and dark depression, and no one knew it. You see, I was doing a great job of hiding it from my family, friends, and colleagues. People had no idea of what I was secretly battling. The person who knew exactly what was happening was, guess who? Me! Since I am a pharmacist, I was aware of the clinical signs and symptoms of depression. If you opened up a textbook and turned to the chapter on major depression, my name and picture may as well have been there. Feelings of sadness and hopelessness most of the day, almost every day, loss of interest in activities, loss of concentration, and thoughts of suicide. I had them ALL!

So many thoughts were racing through my head. So what do I do now? How do I get through this and take my life back? I've worked so hard to get to this point. My family had sacrificed so much for me to go away to college and pharmacy school. I can't let them down. This would break their hearts. My mom and little sister would be devastated. I don't want to die. How do I go on?

Acknowledging that there is a problem is the first step to recovering from anything. Fortunately, I was in a place of acceptance. As a healthcare provider, my next step was to do what I was trained to do if I encountered a person who was having thoughts of suicide: seek help from a trained professional as soon as possible. For me, that was my physician. I picked up the phone one evening and called her. The call went like this:

Me: Hi Doc. This is Jamie.

MD: Hi Jamie. I'm surprised to hear from you this evening. Is everything okay?

Me: Things aren't going so well. I can't eat or sleep. I can't stop crying. I am so sad.

MD: How long has this been going on?

Me: This has been going on for about two months.

MD: Have you had thoughts about harming yourself?

Me: Thoughts of harming myself? (Pause)

MD: Jamie, have you had thoughts about suicide?

Me: (No response. Long pause. Deep breath. In that moment, I had a choice. Do I tell the truth or do I continue to hide it? I decided to say yes.) Yes, I have.

MD: Have you tried to act on those thoughts?

Me: No, I haven't.

MD: When was the last time you had those thoughts?

Me: A few weeks ago.

MD: Okay. I'd like you to come by my office first thing in the morning.

Me: Okay, I will come by the office in the morning.

MD: Will you be okay tonight?

Me: Yes, I will be okay.

MD: I look forward to seeing you in the morning.

Me: I look forward to seeing you too.

That night, I was able to get a few hours of sleep. I arrived for my appointment feeling optimistic that my doctor would get me back on the right track. She listened while I brought her up to speed on everything that had happened and why I was depressed. I had relocated my life and career to be with him. We had talked about engagement rings. I had a feeling he was seeing other people, but I couldn't prove it—until a baby appeared that wasn't mine. I let it all out. She ended the appointment with her plan. I knew what was coming next. As I expected, she took out her prescription pad to write a prescription and also gave me a bag of samples of an antidepressant.

Armed with a Prescription and a Plan

I was excited to begin the journey to get my life back. How ironic was that? The person who manages medication therapy was now receiving medication therapy. I understood that it would take about three weeks for the medication to take effect, so I started taking the samples right away. I was fully aware that this was going to be a process and not a quick fix.

Five days in, the unthinkable happened. I started experiencing side effects like severe headaches, nausea, and dry mouth. Wanting to be a "good patient," I kept taking it. I was determined not to be one of those people that just didn't want to take their medication. On day seven, I called my doctor to report what I was experiencing, and we agreed for me to keep taking it but at a lower dose. That didn't help either. Three

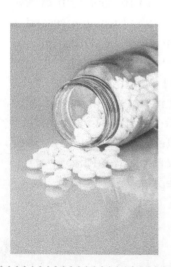

more days passed, and I was still experiencing the side effects. So now what do I do?

Here is where the pharmacist in me got involved. I started evaluating all the clinical options. My doctor could prescribe other medications to treat the side effects that the antidepressant was causing. I could gradually decrease the dose of this medication over several days to safely taper me off of it. From there, I could start taking an antidepressant from a different therapeutic class and slowly increase the dose as tolerated. Ahhhhhh! Clearly, this is where the lines of Jamie the person and Jamie the pharmacist got blurred. I asked myself, *what the hell am I going to do now?*

An Alternative Strategy

As fate would have it, a coworker of mine joined a new gym and gave me a free pass to try it out for a few days. She had no idea what I was secretly battling. I was too embarrassed to tell her. So off to the gym I went— purely out of obligation on the first day. At that time, my only reason for going was so that I didn't appear ungrateful for her kind gesture. Quite honestly, I didn't expect a few visits to the gym to make any difference at all. I didn't have a goal that I was trying to reach. I wasn't focused on fitting into a dress for a special occasion or a swimsuit for a vacation. Interestingly, I went a second day and then a third day in a row.

On my last free pass day, the gym manager informed me of a limited-time promotion to deeply discount the monthly membership fee for new members. Of course I fell for the sales pitch and purchased a membership. No shade. It was a great strategy: offer something of value for FREE and then make an offer that speaks to the needs of the customer. This was sales 101 in action, ya'll. My decision was based on the fact that during those hours in the gym, I didn't feel sad. I let the treadmill, elliptical, and dumb bells feel the wrath of my anger and other negative emotions.

From that point on, I went to the gym every damn day (except Sundays). The gym became my therapy. And guess what happened? The endorphins released from the exercise stabilized my mood; the sadness and anxiety began to decrease. My appetite came

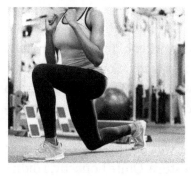

back. I was able to sleep again. I started ear hustling (listening to) the conversations of some of the gym regulars about their habits outside the gym. They talked about magazines

they read and recipes they tried, so I started reading about healthy eating and implementing what I was learning. Food became my medicine. These lifestyle changes LITERALLY saved my life! I looked like my old self again, but honey, I didn't feel like her. I felt better than ever! The Lifestyle Pharmacist was born!

NOTES

NOTES

NOTES

···

The Busy Woman's 21-Day Guide to Clean Eating
PART 2

···

The Truth About Clean Eating

Unlocking the Facts on Fats

Cutting the Salt

Kicking the Sugar Addiction

Fresh Flavors and Aromas

The Truth About Clean Eating

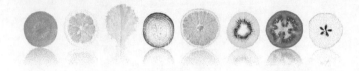

Your eating habits form the foundation of the lifestyle you live. This lifestyle can work for you or against you, and quite frankly, the CHOICE IS YOURS. I am not into doom-and-gloom statistics, but reality checks are sometimes necessary. In the Unites States, a life-style of poor eating habits and drastically reduced levels of physical activity has pushed us over the cliff. While Americans are enjoying a longer lifespan due to advancements in medical technology and innovative treatments, rates of preventable chronic diseases are increasing at alarming rates.

According to the Centers for Disease Control (CDC), "about half of all American adults have one or more preventable chronic diseases, many of which are related to poor quality eating patterns and physical inactivity. These include cardiovascular disease, high blood pressure, type 2 diabetes, some cancers, and poor bone health. More than two-thirds of adults and nearly one-third of children and youth are overweight or obese."[1] The development of these preventable conditions can create a domino effect of health complications. Does any of this sound familiar? Amputations, dialysis, stroke, heart attack, blindness, and arthritis are just a handful of health-related problems brought on by how we treat our bodies. I'm quite sure that you have a friend or family member whose life was cut short or has become less enjoyable because of a preventable health condition. The truth is, NO ONE is exempt! Preventable disease doesn't discriminate. It affects the young and old, middle class and wealthy, African American, Asian, Caucasian, and Latino.

This reality hit me like a ton of bricks early in my career. One day at the hospital, I met a young man while making my rounds on the floor. He was on my list of patients to educate about a medication he was taking. I knocked on the door, introduced myself, and asked if I could talk to him about a new medication he had started taking in the hospital. He agreed, so I sat down and went through the information he needed to know to safely take this medication once he was discharged from the hospital. He listened to what I had to say and then, with a straight face, told me to go get the real pharmacist because I was too young to be one. He was just a few years older than me, by the way. I thought he was serious until he burst into laughter. Relieved that he was joking, I started laughing too. After that, he told me that this time when he goes home, he would take his medication, eat better, and show up for his appointments at the diabetes clinic.

A few hours passed, and I heard a dreaded overhead announcement that a patient was in cardiac arrest on my floor! As the pharmacist on duty, it was my responsibility to go to the bedside and assist with medications. As I ran toward the room where the arrest was happening, I realized that it was the patient I had shared the laughs with. The team did everything possible to bring him back, but unfortunately, it wasn't enough. I was devastated. We were just laughing, and now he was gone. He was 33 years old.

Your health and your quality of life depends on your daily lifestyle habits. There is evidence that shows that healthy eating coupled with physical activity maintain health and prevent or delay the onset of chronic diseases. Everything matters—your snacks, the type of beverages you drink, the foods you eat, the amount of exercise you get, and even the amount of sleep you get at night—they all impact your overall health. The way you eat directly impacts the way you look, how you feel, and most importantly, how you LIVE. The amazing thing is that with the right tools and a personal commitment, you can live a fabulous and fulfilled life.

You may be wondering, "What the heck is eating clean, and what does it have to do with me?" Clean eating is NOT a diet. It represents a lifestyle centered on eating foods in their most natural form. They are foods that have not been chemically modified during the manufacturing process. Simply put, clean eating means:

- No processed foods
- No junk foods
- No fast foods
- No frozen meals
- No boxed meals
- No canned meals

You should eat clean because proper nutrition and health are closely linked. It is nearly impossible to have one without the other. Here is a short list of the benefits of clean eating [14,15]:

- Promotes overall health
- Provides safe and lasting weight loss and weight maintenance
- Regulates your blood glucose, cholesterol, and blood pressure
- Improves your mood
- Promotes more restful sleep
- Reduces hunger and self-deprivation

Unlocking the Facts on Fats

To eat fat or not to eat fat is the question for many people wanting to lose weight or even maintain their desired weight. Fat is high in calories, so many people believe that a healthy diet must contain little to no fat. That is not true. In fact, fat is essential for proper functioning of your body. Cutting out all fat from your diet may cause you to become deficient in essential fatty acids and also the fat-soluble vitamins A, D, E, and K.

What *is* true is that certain types of fat have been linked to the development of cardiovascular disease. The key is knowing which types of fat are good for you and which are bad for you. The main takeaway is that fats are not created equal. Research suggests that healthy fats should be a part of your lifestyle while unhealthy fats should be avoided. I bet you're wondering what the difference is so you can be sure to eat the right type.

There are several types of fat, some of which have long, complicated names, so I understand that it may get confusing. No worries—I'm going to give you an overview on fats so that you include the right type in your diet.

Harmful Fats

There are two types of harmful dietary fats:

The first is **saturated fat**. This is the bad fat that you should avoid overconsuming. Saturated fats are linked to causing heart attacks and strokes because they raise the level of LDL cholesterol in your blood-

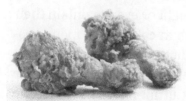

stream. Saturated fats do play a role in the body for proper functioning, but the body makes what it needs naturally. This means there is no need for you to include them in your diet. Your body has this covered without your help. Foods that come to mind for being loaded with saturated fat are foods that contain meat or meat and cheese, such as pizza, burgers, and tacos, to name a few. Fried foods make the naughty list too because they often contain the animal skin and are fried in oils that are high in saturated fat. Other foods include:

- Fatty cuts of beef
- Pork and pork fat
- Poultry with the skin on
- Beef fat
- Lard
- Heavy cream
- Butter
- Cheese
- Products made from whole milk

Trans fat is the second type of fat that should be avoided. Trans fats are created during the production of processed foods and snacks that we eat. These fats are created in a food processing method that adds hydrogen particles to the oil that is an ingredient in the food product. This hydrogenation step is done to make the oil more stable so that the food product tastes better and has a longer shelf life. These oils can also be heated to high temperatures for deep frying foods, and they are inexpensive. That sounds good, right?

That is great for the food manufacturer, but it's bad for you. Here's why: Adding the hydrogen particle to the oil changes it from a liquid to a solid. The problem is that these fats have been shown to increase levels of the bad LDL cholesterol and decrease levels of the good HDL cholesterol. These cholesterol alterations increase your risk of cardiovascular disease, stroke, and the development of type 2 diabetes. So it's important to realize that some crackers, cookies, snack foods, vegetable shortenings, sticks of margarine, frozen foods, and fried foods are loaded with trans fat.

There are a few simple ways to spot trans fats in foods. Look at the food label to see if you see the words "trans fat" or "partially hydrogenated oil" listed as an ingredient. Select foods that state on the label that they contain 0 grams of trans fat and no partially hydrogenated oil. This is important to know because the primary dietary source for trans fats in processed food is "partially hydrogenated oils." The serious health consequences of eating foods containing trans fats have been well studied. According to the American Heart Association, "in November 2013, the U.S. Food and Drug Administration (FDA) made a preliminary determination that partially hydrogenated oils are no longer generally recognized as safe in human food."[2,5]

Healthy Fats

There are three types of fats that provide health benefits from their consumption: monounsaturated fats, polyunsaturated fats, and omega-3 fatty acids. Of course I will give you the health scoop and tell you how to recognize these healthy fats. Studies show that eating foods rich in **mono and polyunsaturated fats** decrease your risk of heart disease by improving cholesterol levels. There is also data showing improved blood glucose control from eating these fats. This is especially beneficial for individuals living with diabetes and prediabetes. Mono and polyunsaturated fats are liquids at room temperature and can be found in the following plant-based oils: peanut oil, corn oil, olive oil, safflower oil, and canola oil. Cooking with them at home and also consuming foods that include them are great for your health.

Omega-3 fatty acids are a type of polyunsaturated fat derived from fish, some nuts, and seeds. Omega-3 fatty acids may be especially beneficial to your heart health as they decrease triglyceride levels, which decrease the risk of coronary artery disease. They also are associated with decreasing inflammation in the body. This can be helpful for people suffering with any illness or disease caused by inflammation. Including foods rich in omega-3 fatty acids in your diet is recommended. Here is a short list of omega-3 containing foods to eat regularly:

- Wild-caught salmon
- Sardines
- Trout
- Anchovies

- Flaxseeds
- Chia seeds
- Sunflower seeds
- Walnuts

Take Home Points

It is important to your long-term health to know the facts on fat!

The newly published 2015–2020 Dietary Guidelines for Americans offers the following recommendations about dietary fat intake[4]:

- Avoid trans fat and partially hydrogenated oils.

- Limit saturated fat intake to less than 10 percent of total daily calories.

- Replace saturated fat with healthier monounsaturated and polyunsaturated fats.

Cutting the Salt

Are your taste buds getting the best of you? Do they call the shots when you sit down at the table to eat? Do they cause you to pile more of certain foods onto your plate while totally ignoring others? I have good news and great news. The good news is that you are not alone. The great news is that you can hit the reset button on your salt-loving taste buds.

I'm not just talking about salt that you shake onto

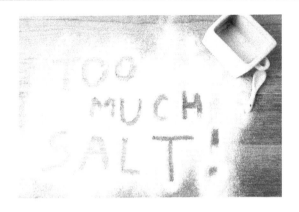

your food. I'm also referring to the high amount of sodium in the restaurant meals, processed foods, and snacks that busy women have grown to rely on. You see, the salt in packaged and processed foods decreases bacterial growth, adds stability to the product so that it has a longer shelf life, and enhances the flavor profile. I'm not suggesting that the restaurant owners and food manufacturers are out to get you. I do, however, want you to be informed and aware of the extremely high amount of salt in those "convenience foods" that you eat for breakfast, lunch, dinner, and snacks.

The average sodium intake in the United States is approximately 3,400 milligrams per day. No big deal? Wrong! That is way over the recommended daily sodium intake amount. According to the 2015–2020 Dietary Guidelines, adults are advised to consume no more than 2,300 milligrams of sodium a day.[8] This maximum daily amount isn't random. It is based on evidence showing that as sodium intake increases, blood pressure also increases. So it comes as no surprise that this persistent overconsumption of sodium is a factor in the development of hypertension or high blood pressure. High blood pressure has been nicknamed the silent killer since it contributes to heart disease and strokes, which are leading causes of death in the United States.

The food industry still has some hard work ahead of it to implement sodium reductions in manufactured foods. So what can you do? You can decrease your intake of these foods by preparing your meals and snacks at home. That way you can be in complete control of what goes in your meals and subsequently inside your body. The food choices we make on a daily basis play a critical role in our health both now and in the future.

Additional tips for limiting sodium intake include:

- Comparing food labels and selecting options with the least amount of sodium.
- Cooking at home using fresh ingredients in their most natural form.
- Limiting how often you eat restaurant food.
- Requesting nutrition information when dining out.

Take Home Points

It is important to your long-term health to know how dietary salt affects your health!

According to the 2015–2020 Dietary Guidelines, adults are advised to consume no more than 2,300 mg of sodium a day.[8]

Two simple ways are to:

- Cook at home using fresh ingredients.

- Decrease your intake of processed foods and restaurant meals.

Kicking the Sugar Addiction

The consumption of excessive amounts of sugar is another challenge faced by many people. It is estimated that an average of 270 calories consumed each day comes from added sugars.[11] This sugar is not just in the form of cakes, pies, brownies, cookies, pastries, and ice cream either. The largest culprit is beverages. Shocked? Think about it like this. Some of your favorite beverages like soft drinks, tea, coffee, energy drinks, sports drinks, flavored water, and juice contain high amounts of sugar. In fact, "beverages account for almost half (47 percent) of all added sugars consumed by the U.S. population." Of that percentage, 25 percent comes from soft drinks alone. So

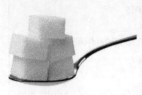

you can understand how the combination of these foods and beverages easily causes individuals to exceed the recommendation that a maximum of 10 percent of calories should come from sugar each day.[11,16]

You may be thinking, what's the problem with eating and drinking sugar? Sugar has been associated with significant health problems. There is data indicating that dietary sugar supports the formation of belly fat. The location of a large amount of fat in the abdominal area is particularly problematic because having a large amount of belly fat increases the risk of cardiovascular disease, insulin resistance, and type 2 diabetes. High amounts of circulating sugar can negatively affect your memory and your brain function. There is a growing body of evidence suggesting that a diet high in sugar may increase the risk for developing Alzheimer's disease and depression.

Perhaps you are not a sweet eater, but a large part of your food is in the form of processed meals and snacks. Well my dear, sugar is a key ingredient in those processed food items. The silver lining is that you can kick your sugar addiction in two simple ways:

1. Cut out the sugary beverages. This simple modification can easily trim 400 to 500 calories form your daily intake. Don't get caught sipping on unnecessary calories. Instead of reaching for

manufactured juices, soft drinks, and specialty coffees, sip on water, unsweetened tea, and low-fat milk instead. This may sound hard, but it can be simple with proper planning and preparation.

2. A lifestyle tip that I live by, and you should adopt, is to drink half your weight in ounces of water every day. Maybe you don't like the taste of water. No worries. Use fresh herbs, fresh or frozen fruit, and freshly squeezed fruit juice to add more flavor to the water. That way, you won't dread drinking water.

Take Home Points

It is important to your long-term health to know how to spot hidden sugars in foods and drinks!

According to the 2015–2020 Dietary Guidelines, adults are advised to consume no more than 10 percent of daily calories as sugar.[11,16]

Three simple strategies are to:

- Minimize your intake of processed foods and snacks that are filled with sugar.

- Make water your beverage of choice.

- Avoid sugary soft drinks, specialty coffees, and manufactured juices.

Fresh Flavors and Aromas

There is a myth that healthy foods are boring and bland. Many people believe that foods that are good for you can't also taste good to you. That simply isn't true. The key to enjoying clean meals is using fresh ingredients and layering the flavors.

The use of fresh herbs and regional spices add an exotic flair to your food. They are a great way to

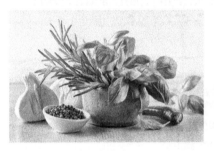

amplify the flavor profile in your clean meals. The great thing is that you don't have to be a trained chef to master flavor mixing. Of course, I have a few tips to share so that you can try this at home. The key is to choose one culinary style for your meal. Then gather three or more signature ingredients from that particular style for incorporation into your meal. Your taste buds won't know what hit them! Your clean meals will be anything but boring and bland.

A few of my favorite culinary styles are Creole, Southern, Thai, Caribbean, Mexican, Italian, and Moroccan. Spoiler alert! I will be sharing some yummy recipes from these styles with you in part 3 of the book, so stay tuned.

Here is the scoop on the key ingredients making up each culinary style[10]:

- Creole: garlic, onion, cayenne pepper, paprika, bell peppers, celery
- Southern: onion, celery, okra, paprika, garlic
- Thai: cilantro, mint, Thai basil, green onion, lime, ginger
- Caribbean: allspice, nutmeg, cinnamon, scotch bonnet pepper
- Mexican: cilantro, cumin, chipotle, lime, cilantro, chili peppers
- Italian: oregano, basil, capers, olives, oranges
- Moroccan: saffron, cumin, lemon, cayenne, cinnamon

You can also kick your clean meals up a notch by adding aromatics and flavor enhancers as you cook and to finish off your dish. Here's how:

Fresh Herbs
- Add fresh herbs to vegetables as they cook.
- Garnish the completed dish with fresh herbs.

Dried Herbs
- Add dried herbs and spices to your carbohydrates as they cook.

Citrus
- Squeeze fresh citrus juice over your protein as it cooks or once plated.

Nuts
- Sprinkle chopped or sliced nuts onto your plate once all the meal components are added.

Onion
- Sauté green vegetables and onion in the skillet together to add sweetness and depth of flavor.

Pan Sauces
- Use the liquid produced from cooking chicken, seafood, and pork as a flavorful sauce.

Garlic Cloves
- When roasting vegetables, include fresh cloves of garlic as a yummy garnish.

Red Pepper Flakes
- Layer additional flavor into proteins by sprinkling them with red pepper flakes as they cook.

Take Home Points

- Clean eating does NOT have to be boring and bland!

- Make your taste buds fall in love with clean eating by adding fresh herbs and exotic spices to your food.

- Choose one culinary style to anchor your meal and use ingredients from that style while cooking each component.

NOTES

NOTES

NOTES

··

The Busy Woman's 21-Day Guide to Clean Eating
PART 3

··

Following the Guide

21 Breakfasts

21 Lunches

21 Dinners

Snack Ideas

Following the Guide

There are a handful of objections busy women give when challenged to make a change in their lifestyle. So let's go ahead and get them out of the way right now. You want to eat healthy and apply these clean eating principles to your lifestyle, but you are too busy to look for recipes. You are overwhelmed at just the thought of stepping out of your regular food routine, and you are afraid that you will do it wrong or you don't have the time to plan meals that follow all of the rules. Deciding what the meals will be, shopping for the ingredients, and then cooking seems impossible. With your job, the kids, your business, sending emails, networking, meeting deadlines, spending time with your spouse or significant other, not to mention making time for friends and family, or even yourself. Ahhhhhhh! You're ready to quit before you even begin.

Will someone just tell you what to buy and what to eat when, and you will do it? Would that be the answer to your frustration and inability to cut the convenient junk food and processed food habit? For someone to grab you by the hand and walk you through every snack and meal for a few weeks? Look no further. That is exactly what I will do for you. I get it. I was you. I was in that exact same state of paralysis and overwhelm, feeling too busy to change my daily eating habits. It's just quicker and easier to order take out for dinner, eat a frozen meal for lunch, and have coffee and a pastry for breakfast.

Worry no more. I, Dr. Jamie, have designed this 21-day clean eating guide for the busy woman. You will learn to "Eat Your Way to Fabulous" in 21 days. You will eat less refined sugars and saturated fats. You will eat more whole grains, lean proteins, and fruits and vegetables. You will drink less sugary beverages and learn to hydrate with water and healthier beverage options. You may even lose a few pounds as a side effect of changing the way you eat. The awesome thing is that this gets you on a path to making healthy eating patterns a part of your daily life, which will produce lasting results. You know what I always say: diets don't work, but lifestyle changes last a lifetime.

Here's how it works. You will eat at least three small meals and two snacks every day for 21 days. And it goes a little something like this: breakfast> snack> lunch> snack> dinner. Oh, you thought you would be hungry? No ma'am. Rule #1 in the #FABSQUAD is to eat REAL FOOD. No hunger is allowed. To make it even easier, the recipes and the schedules are provided here. This guide tells you what to eat and when to eat. All the homework and research have been done for you. Simply follow the recipes and the food schedule, and you will be well on your way to looking and feeling FABULOUS!

Daily Meal Schedule

MEAL	TIME
Breakfast	6:30–7:30 a.m.
Snack	10:00 a.m.
Lunch	12:30 p.m.
Snack	3:30 p.m.
Dinner	6:30–7:30 p.m.

21 Breakfasts

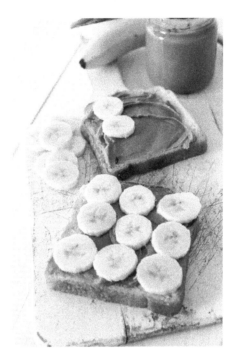

While you were sleeping, your body was FASTING. It's time to break the fast with breakfast. Clean, delicious morning fuel coming right up!

General Principle: Simple recipes are ideal for fast-paced weekday mornings. Save the more involved recipes for weekend mornings where you can spend a little more time in the kitchen.

All recipes are single serving unless noted otherwise.

Weekday Recipes

Fruit and Cottage Cheese Breakfast Parfait[18]

Ingredients:

½ cup cottage cheese
¼ cup chopped pineapple
¼ cup sliced strawberries
3 tablespoons of whole granola

How to Make:

1. In a tall glass, alternate layers of cottage cheese and fruit (three layers each).
2. Top with whole granola grain and enjoy.

Farmhouse Stack[18]

<u>Ingredients:</u>

½ cup spinach (frozen or fresh)
1 egg (scrambled or sunny side up)
1 slice of Swiss cheese
1 whole wheat English muffin or slice of whole wheat toast

<u>How to Make:</u>

1. Steam the spinach in a nonstick skillet or microwave safe bowl and place on a saucer.
2. Place 1 slice of low-fat Swiss cheese on top of the spinach.
3. Cook 1 large egg (anyway you like).
4. Place the egg on top of the cheese.
5. Serve with 1 whole wheat English muffin or slice of whole wheat toast.

Grown Folk's Fruit Cocktail

<u>Ingredients per bowl:</u>

½ cup store-bought sugar-free fruit cocktail packed in water, drained
⅓ cup coconut flakes
½ cup vanilla Greek yogurt
¼ cup chopped almonds

<u>How to Make:</u>

1.   Place the fruit cocktail in a small bowl.
2.   Top the fruit with Greek yogurt.
3.   Sprinkle the coconut flakes on top of the yogurt.
4.   Sprinkle the chopped almonds over the coconut flakes.

Garden Egg Scramble[19]

<u>Ingredients:</u>

2 large beaten eggs
¼ cup fresh or frozen spinach
1 diced roma tomato
¼ cup of sliced mushrooms
¼ cup shredded mozzarella cheese
1 teaspoon of black pepper
1 tablespoon olive oil
1 pinch of kosher salt

<u>How to Make:</u>

1. Heat olive oil in a small nonstick skillet.
2. Add vegetables and cook until softened.
3. Add black pepper and pinch of kosher salt (if desired).
4. Add eggs and scramble them with the vegetables.
5. Add mozzarella cheese and remove from heat.

Whole Wheat Toast with Almond Butter and Bananas

Ingredients:

1 banana, sliced
2 pieces of whole wheat toast
2 tablespoons almond butter
½ teaspoon chia seeds, optional

How to Make:

1. Spread 1 tablespoon of almond butter onto each slice of toast.

2. Add ½ sliced banana to each slice of toast.

3. Finish each slice of toast with a sprinkle of chia seeds.

Greek Yogurt Bowl

Ingredients:

1 cup vanilla Greek yogurt
½ cup mixed blueberries, strawberries, raspberries (you can buy frozen and allow to unthaw in the fridge overnight)
⅓ cup granola

How to Make:

1. Place the Greek yogurt in a small bowl.
2. Top with the mixed berries.
3. Finish with a sprinkle of granola.

Loaded Cantaloupe[20]

Servings: 2; Portion: ½ cantaloupe

Ingredients:

1 small cantaloupe, cut in half
½ cup Greek vanilla yogurt
⅓ cup blueberries (fresh or frozen)
Sprinkle of granola

How to Make:

1. Cut a cantaloupe in half and scoop out the seeds.
2. Place yogurt inside the center of 1 piece and set the other half aside.
3. Top with blueberries and granola.

Green Breakfast Smoothie[21]

Ingredients:

1 cup fresh spinach
1 cup almond milk
1 green apple, sliced
1 banana
½ cup green grapes

How to Make:

1. Add spinach and almond milk to a blender and blend well.
2. Add the apple, banana, and grapes and blend again.
3. Add a teaspoon of flaxseed, chia seeds, almond butter or protein powder and blend once more (optional).
4. Serve in your favorite glass or in a blender bottle to take on the go.

Berry Bliss Breakfast Smoothie[22]

<u>Ingredients:</u>

1 cup mixed frozen raspberries, strawberries, and blueberries
½ cup vanilla Greek yogurt
1 banana
2 scoops protein powder (whey or plant-based)
1 cup almond milk
1 teaspoon honey to sweeten, optional

<u>How to Make:</u>

1. Add the ingredients to a blender and blend well.
2. Serve in your favorite glass or in a blender bottle to take on the go.

Baked Egg and Bacon Avocado Boats[23]

<u>Ingredients:</u>

1 avocado, halved
2 eggs, uncooked
2 slices turkey bacon, crumbled
2 tablespoons fresh salsa
¼ teaspoon salt and freshly ground pepper, if desired
¼ teaspoon cayenne pepper
1 tablespoon olive oil

<u>How to Make:</u>

1. Preheat oven to 425 degrees.
2. Cut avocado in half and remove the pit.
3. Place avocados on an oiled baking pan.
4. Crack 1 egg into each avocado half, season with salt, black pepper, and cayenne pepper.
5. Bake uncovered for about 15 minutes until entire egg is cooked through.
6. Garnish each avocado with crumbled bacon and salsa.
7. Serve with 1 piece of whole wheat toast.

Make-Ahead Chia Pudding and Fruit[24]

<u>Ingredients:</u>

1 cup coconut or almond milk
2 cups chia seeds
½ teaspoon vanilla extract
¼ cup honey (maple syrup or agave can be used as sweeteners)
4 strawberries, sliced

<u>How to Make:</u>

1. Pour all the ingredients into a glass jar.
2. Secure the lid and shake the jar to combine the ingredients.
3. Place jar in the refrigerator overnight to gel.
4. For blended/smooth version: Place all ingredients in blender and blend on high for 1 to 2 minutes until completely smooth.
5. Serve in a bowl topped with sliced strawberries and enjoy.

Spiced Avocado Toast[25]

<u>Ingredients:</u>

1 avocado, mashed with a squeeze of lime juice
2 slices whole wheat toast
Sea salt and red pepper flakes to taste

<u>How to Make:</u>

1. Spread mashed avocado onto each slice of whole wheat toast.
2. Season with a pinch of sea salt and red pepper flakes.

Rainbow Smoothie Bowl[26]

<u>Ingredients:</u>

1 cup frozen mango
1 cup frozen pineapple
1 packet of frozen dragon fruit puree
1 banana, sliced
½ cup coconut milk
1 scoop protein powder (whey or plant-based)
2 fresh strawberries, sliced
Granola, optional topping
Coconut flakes, optional topping

<u>How to Make:</u>

1. Combine the mango, pineapple, dragon fruit, ½ of sliced banana, coconut milk, and protein powder in the blender and blend until smooth (save a little mango to use as a topping)
2. Pour smoothie into a bowl.
3. Top with sliced strawberries, sliced bananas, mango, coconut flakes, and granola or whole grain cereal.

Make-Ahead Just Peachy Overnighter Oatmeal[27]

<u>Ingredients:</u>

½ cup oats (rolled or steel cut)
½ cup coconut milk
1 tablespoon honey
1 teaspoon coconut flakes
1 tablespoon chopped pecans
1 fresh peach, chopped

<u>How to Make:</u>

1. Add oats and milk to a mason jar.
2. Add a layer of peaches, almonds, and coconut.
3. Drizzle honey on top and place the lid on the jar.
4. Refrigerate overnight.

Savory Grapefruit[28]

<u>Ingredients:</u>

1 grapefruit, halved
¼ teaspoon cinnamon
¼ teaspoon nutmeg
½ teaspoon brown sugar

<u>How to Make:</u>

1. Preheat the oven to broil.
2. Cut the grapefruit in half. Loosen the fruit by going around the edges with a knife where the fruit meets the peel.
3. Sprinkle cinnamon, nutmeg, and brown sugar over grapefruit halves.
4. Place grapefruit on a baking sheet and broil until the sugar browns (about 6 minutes).
5. Remove from oven and allow to cool for 3 minutes before eating.

Weekend Recipes

Whole Wheat and Banana Silver Dollar Pancakes[29]

Ingredients:

1 ripe banana
2 tablespoons whole wheat flour
1 large egg, beaten
½ teaspoon of baking powder
1 teaspoon of honey
½ teaspoon of nutmeg
½ teaspoon of cinnamon
Optional pancake toppings: 2 tablespoons of part-skim ricotta cheese, ¼ cup fresh blueberries, 1 teaspoon of walnuts, and 1 teaspoon of honey.

How to Make:

1. Mash a banana with a fork until smooth.
2. Add the dry ingredients, honey, and egg to the mashed banana and whisk well.
3. Heat a large nonstick skillet over medium-high heat.
4. Spoon the batter into the skillet for 3, silver dollar-sized pancakes
5. Wait until bubbles cover the tops and then flip the pancakes over (about 2 minutes).
6. Cook 1 to 2 minutes on this side until brown.
7. Top with any of the optional pancake toppings.

Loaded Quinoa Muffins[30]

Ingredients:

1 cup cooked quinoa
2 eggs, beaten
½ cup shredded zucchini
½ cup chopped turkey breast (whole breast or slices)
1 chopped green onion
Kosher salt and black pepper to taste
1 cup grated cheddar cheese

How to Make:

1. Preheat oven to 350 degrees.
2. Mix the ingredients together in a bowl.
3. Spray muffin tins with cooking spray.
4. Spoon the filling into the top of each muffin cup.
5. Bake for 25 to 30 minutes until the edges turn golden brown.
6. Cool in the muffin tin for 5 minutes before removing.

Coconut, Almond, Cranberry Breakfast Bars[31]

Ingredients:

⅓ cup almond butter
⅓ cup honey
1 tablespoon olive oil
1 teaspoon vanilla extract
½ teaspoon kosher salt
1 cup puffed wheat cereal
⅓ cup chopped almonds
⅓ cup unsweetened coconut
1 cup rolled oats
⅔ cup dried cranberries

How to Make:

1. Preheat oven to 350 degrees.
2. Generously spray a cooking sheet with cooking spray.
3. In a microwave safe bowl, combine almond butter, honey, olive oil, salt, and vanilla extract.
4. Microwave until mixture becomes bubbly (about 1 minute).
5. In a bowl, combine oats, puffed wheat, dried cranberries, almonds, and coconut.
6. Pour the almond butter mixture over the oat mixture and combine well.
7. Press the mixture into the cooking sheet.
8. Bake for 10 minutes.
9. Remove from oven and allow to completely cool before cutting.

Huevos Rancheros Breakfast Bowl[32]

Servings: 4; Portion: 1 bowl

Ingredients:

4 Italian hot turkey sausages removed from the casings
1 can low sodium black beans (rinsed and drained)
1 can low sodium diced tomatoes
1½ teaspoon cumin
½ teaspoon ancho chili powder (or chipotle chili powder to substitute)
1 tablespoon lime juice
4 large eggs
¼ cup chopped cilantro
1 lime cut into wedges
1 sliced avocado
1 tablespoon canola oil
Queso fresco cheese

How to Make:

1. Heat a nonstick skillet over medium heat and cook the meat until browned. Break it into pieces with the back of a wooden spoon.

2. Stir in the beans, tomatoes with juice, cumin, and chili powder.

3. Bring to a boil; then reduce to low heat and simmer until thickened.

4. Remove from heat and stir in lime juice.

5. Heat 1 tablespoon canola oil in a nonstick skillet over medium heat.

6. Crack each egg into the skillet and let cook for 1 minute. Flip them with a spatula, turn the heat to low, cover skillet, and cook 5 minutes, or until egg is the

desired texture (longer for hard, shorter for soft).

7. To serve, spoon the meat and bean mixture into a bowl.

8. Add an egg.

9. Crumble 2 teaspoons of queso fresco cheese on top.

10. Garnish with 1 teaspoon of cilantro, a lime wedge, and 2 avocado slices.

Peanut Butter and Chocolate Protein Waffles[33]

<u>Ingredients:</u>

1 scoop protein powder (whey or plant based)
1 tablespoon almond flour
1 teaspoon baking powder
1 egg
3 tablespoons water
1 teaspoon canola oil
¼ cup dark chocolate chips
½ sliced banana
2 tablespoons warmed peanut butter

<u>How to Make:</u>

1. Preheat waffle iron.
2. Combine protein powder, almond flour, baking powder, and egg into a bowl.
3. Blend well with a hand mixer or whisk.
4. Create a thick pancake batter like consistency by adding water one tablespoon at a time to the bowl of dry ingredients.
5. Fold the chocolate chips into the batter.
6. Spray waffle iron with cooking spray.
7. Spoon batter onto the waffle iron.
8. Cook waffle until crispy and golden brown.
9. Serve with drizzle of warm peanut butter and top waffles with banana slices.

Turkey Sausage BrEGGfast Skillet[34]

Servings: 4; Portion: 1 bowl

Ingredients:

1 tablespoon olive oil
2 cloves garlic, minced
1 pound turkey breakfast sausage
1 can fire roasted diced tomatoes
⅓ cup basil pesto, store bought
4 large eggs
½ teaspoon kosher salt
½ teaspoon black pepper
¼ teaspoon onion powder
½ teaspoon Italian seasoning
¼ cup low-fat mozzarella cheese, grated

How to Make:

1. Heat olive oil in a skillet over medium-high heat.
2. Add turkey sausage, garlic, salt, pepper, and onion powder, and cook until brown.
3. Add tomatoes and basil pesto and stir to combine.
4. Reduce to medium heat and simmer for 2 minutes.
5. Crack open the eggs on top of the sausage and tomato mixture.
6. Season with a pinch of salt and pepper.
7. Cover and cook 7 to 9 minutes or until the eggs reach the desired consistency.
8. Remove the lid and sprinkle with mozzarella.

21 Lunches

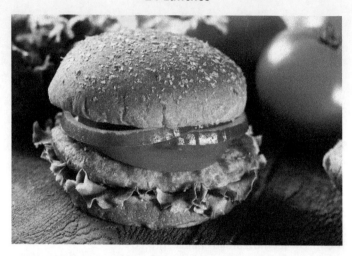

Some of the lunch recipes will put your dinner left-overs to good use. Smart, right? I got the memo. You're very busy. No unnecessary cooking allowed on my watch!

General Principle: Repurposing dinner leftovers into flavorful lunches saves time during the week and on the weekend too.

All recipes are single serving unless noted otherwise.

<u>*Recipes Using Dinner Leftovers*</u>

Salmon Salad[35]

<u>Ingredients:</u>

½ cup flaked salmon
1 tablespoon olive oil
1 tablespoon lemon juice
2 sliced Kalamata olives
1 teaspoon red onion, finely chopped
1 teaspoon fresh parsley, chopped
1 teaspoon capers, chopped

<u>How to Make:</u>

1. Combine salmon, oil, lemon juice, olives, red onion, parsley, and capers in a small bowl.
2. Serve with 4 whole wheat crackers and a ½ cup of grapes.

Cook's Note: This is a great way to use leftover salmon.

Moroccan Quinoa Salad[36]

<u>Ingredients:</u>

2 cups water
1 cup quinoa
1 cup leftover Moroccan cucumber salad

<u>How to Make:</u>

1. Bring the water to a boil and add the quinoa.
2. Reduce the heat to low, cover and simmer for 15 to 20 minutes until tender and until most of the liquid has been absorbed.
3. Strain and rinse well with cold water, being sure to remove all moisture.
4. Once dry, transfer the quinoa to a large bowl.
5. Add the leftover Moroccan cucumber salad and toss well.
6. Add a pinch of kosher salt and black pepper if desired.

Cook's Note: This is a great way to use leftover Moroccan cucumber salad.

Shrimp Salad[37]

Servings: 2; Portion: 1 bowl

<u>Salad Ingredients:</u>

1 bag of chopped romaine lettuce
8 sautéed shrimp, cut in half
½ cup cherry tomatoes, cut in half
Dressing Ingredients:
2½ tablespoons fresh lemon juice
⅛ teaspoon kosher salt
1½ tablespoons olive oil
½ teaspoon whole grain Dijon mustard

<u>How to Make:</u>

1. Add the lettuce and tomatoes to a large bowl.
2. Place the sautéed shrimp on top.
3. For the dressing, add kosher salt, lemon juice, olive oil, and mustard in a bowl, stirring with a whisk.
4. Drizzle the dressing on top of the salad and toss to mix.

Cook's Note: This is a great way to use leftover shrimp scampi.

Cheeseburger Salad[38]

Servings: 2; Portion: 1 bowl

<u>Ingredients:</u>

2 turkey burger patties, diced
1 medium red onion, sliced
1 bag of chopped romaine lettuce
1 cup fresh tomato, chopped
¾ cup reduced-fat cheddar cheese, shredded
⅓ cup olive oil mayonnaise
¼ cup ketchup
2 tablespoons water
1 teaspoon olive oil
1 cup plain or flavored reduced-fat kettle-cooked potato chips

<u>How to Make:</u>

1. Heat 1 teaspoon of olive oil in a nonstick skillet over medium heat.
2. Add onions to pan and cook until tender.
3. Add diced turkey burgers to the pan with the onions to rewarm them and then remove from heat.
4. In a large bowl, combine romaine, burger pieces, onion, tomato, and cheese.
5. For the dressing, whisk together mayonnaise, ketchup, and 2 tablespoons water in a small bowl.
6. Drizzle dressing over salad.
7. Lightly crush kettle chips and sprinkle over salad for a crunchy topping.

Cook's Note: This is a great way to use leftover turkey burgers.

Peruvian Chicken Salad Sandwich[39]

Ingredients:

1 cup leftover Peruvian chicken, shredded
⅓ cup olive oil mayonnaise
½ cup plain Greek yogurt
1 tablespoon lime juice
1 teaspoon honey
¼ teaspoon paprika
¼ teaspoon salt
¼ teaspoon black pepper
¼ teaspoon cumin
1 cup red onion, finely chopped
1 cup red seedless grapes, halved
½ cup roasted almonds, coarsely chopped
2 slices whole wheat bread
1 piece of green leaf lettuce

How to Make:

1. Whisk mayonnaise, yogurt, cumin, lime juice, honey, paprika, salt, and pepper in a large bowl.
2. Add chicken, onion, grapes, and almonds and stir gently to combine.
3. Season to taste with a pinch of kosher salt and black pepper.
4. Place chicken salad on a slice of bread and top with a piece of lettuce and another piece of bread.
5. Serve with half of a sliced apple.

Cook's Note: This is a great way to use leftover Peruvian chicken.

Fresh Harvest Salad[40]

Servings: 2; Portion: 1 bowl

<u>Ingredients:</u>

1 bag mixed greens salad
1 cup shredded orange oven roasted chicken
1 Gala apple, cut into chunks
¼ cup walnuts
½ cup dried cranberries
¼ cup crumbled blue cheese

<u>How to Make:</u>

1. Combine the ingredients into a plastic storage container.
2. Place the cover on it and shake to mix the salad.
3. Serve with 1 teaspoon light raspberry walnut vinaigrette dressing.

Cook's Note: This is a great way to use leftover oven roasted orange chicken.

Blackened Catfish Sandwich[41]

Ingredients:

1 blackened catfish fillet
1 large tomato slice
1 piece green leaf lettuce
1 whole wheat bun
½ cup coleslaw
1 teaspoon homemade tartar sauce

Tartar Sauce Ingredients:
2 tablespoons reduced fat mayonnaise
2 tablespoons plain Greek yogurt
½ tablespoon sweet pickle relish
1 teaspoon garlic powder

How to Make Tartar Sauce:

1. Mix the ingredients together in a small bowl.
2. Place in a sealed container and refrigerate until ready to use.

How to Make Blackened Catfish Sandwich:

1. Place 1 warmed blackened catfish fillet on a whole wheat bun.
2. Garnish with a piece of green leaf lettuce a slice of tomato.
3. Smear ½ teaspoon of tartar sauce on the top bun and place it on the sandwich.
4. Serve with ½ cup of leftover coleslaw.

Cook's Note: This is a great way to use leftover blackened catfish and leftover coleslaw.

Loaded Greek Pita[42]

Ingredients:

½ cup chopped romaine lettuce
1 whole wheat pita
2 tablespoons crumbled feta cheese
½ cucumber, sliced
1 small tomato, sliced
2 tablespoons Greek salad dressing, store bought
3 leftover lamb kabobs, cut in half

How to Make:

1. Take a pita and stuff the inside with lettuce.
2. Add the sliced tomato and cucumber.
3. Add the cheese and warm lamb kabobs.
4. Drizzle the Greek dressing on top.

Cook's Note: This is a great way to used leftover lamb kabobs.

Quick Cooked Lunches

Chicken Hummus Wrap [43]

<u>Ingredients:</u>

3 tablespoons hummus, store bought
1 whole wheat wrap
1 sliced baked skinless chicken breast
3 avocado slices
2 tomato slices
½ cup shredded lettuce

<u>How to Make:</u>

1. Lay the whole wheat wrap on a flat surface and spread the hummus in the center.
2. Add a layer of romaine lettuce to the center.
3. Add the sliced chicken.
4. Add the sliced tomato.
5. Roll it up and cut in half (a toothpick can be used to hold the wrap in place).

Black Bean Quesadillas and Black Bean Corn Salsa[44,45]

Servings: 2; Portion: 3 wedges

<u>Black Bean Corn Salsa Ingredients:</u>

½ cup canned black beans, rinsed and drained
½ cup canned whole kernel corn, rinsed and drained
½ cup fresh pico de gallo (store bought)
2 tablespoons chopped cilantro
1 tablespoon lime juice
½ teaspoon chili powder
½ teaspoon garlic powder
¼ teaspoon kosher salt
Black Bean Quesadilla Ingredients:
1 cup canned black beans, rinsed and drained
½ cup diced tomato
2 whole wheat tortillas
½ cup shredded low-fat cheddar cheese
1 small red bell pepper, cut into thin strips
1 teaspoon garlic, minced
1 teaspoon cumin
2 teaspoons chili powder
2 teaspoons olive oil

<u>How to Make Black Bean Corn Salsa:</u>

1. Add the black beans, corn, and pico de gallo to a bowl.
2. Add the chopped cilantro, lime juice, chili powder, garlic powder, salt, and mix well.

<u>How to Make Black Bean Quesadillas:</u>

1. Preheat the oven to 400 degrees.
2. Mix the black beans, cumin, and chili powder in a bowl.

3. Mash the beans with a fork until a creamy consistency.

4. Add the olive oil, red bell pepper, and garlic to a nonstick skillet and cook until tender.

5. Place the tortillas on a flat surface and spread the black beans on one half of the tortilla.

6. Place the bell pepper on top of the black beans.

7. Sprinkle a layer of cheese over the bell peppers.

8. Close the tortilla by folding the other half over the side with the filling.

9. Spray a baking sheet with cooking spray and bake the quesadilla on each side for 4 minutes until the cheese melts and they are heated through.

10. Cut each quesadilla into 3 pieces.

Turkey Burgers

Servings: 4; Portion: 1 turkey burger

Ingredients:

1 pound package of ground turkey
1 bag frozen sweet potato fries
Green leaf lettuce
Sliced tomato
Whole wheat buns
1 teaspoon kosher salt
Black pepper
¼ cup shredded cheddar cheese

How to Make Turkey Burgers:

1. Form the ground turkey into patties and season with salt and pepper.
2. In the meantime, heat the oven to 425 degrees and place frozen sweet potato fries on an oiled baking sheet.
3. Once patties are cooked through, remove from the heat.
4. Place the cheese on the remaining patties and cover to melt the cheese.
5. Assemble the sandwich by placing a turkey patty on the bun and add the lettuce and tomato.
6. Serve with 1 serving of sweet potatoes fries.

Cook's Note: Leftover turkey burgers (2 patties) can be used to make the Cheeseburger Salad lunch recipe.

Turkey, Cucumber, and Tomato Sandwich Minis[46]

<u>Ingredients:</u>

1 cucumber, sliced
Turkey breast, thinly sliced
1 roma tomato, sliced
Black pepper

<u>How to Make:</u>

1. Slice the cucumber into rounds to use as the top and bottoms of the mini sandwiches.
2. Place a piece of sliced turkey and tomato on top of a cucumber.
3. Season with a pinch of black pepper and place a cucumber on top.
4. Use a toothpick to hold each mini sandwich in place.
5. Serve 5 mini sandwiches with ½ cup of diced melon.

Caprese Pasta Salad[47]

<u>Ingredients:</u>

1 cup wheat bowtie pasta
3 tablespoons basil pesto (store bought)
1 tablespoon olive oil
¼ teaspoon garlic powder
¼ teaspoon black pepper
1 teaspoon Italian seasoning
½ teaspoon kosher salt
½ cup grape tomatoes, halved
½ cup fresh mozzarella balls, halved

<u>How to Make:</u>

1. Bring a pot of water to a boil and cook the pasta until tender yet firm (about 8 minutes).
2. Drain the pasta.
3. Mix pasta, pesto, olive oil, salt, garlic, Italian seasoning, and black pepper in a bowl.
4. Toss to coat and fold in the tomatoes and mozzarella.

Bacon Avocado Lettuce and Tomato Sandwich[48]

Ingredients:

4 slices turkey bacon
1 avocado, mashed
2 pieces of green leaf lettuce
1 tomato, sliced

How to Make:

1. Cook the turkey bacon until crisp.
2. In a bowl, mash an avocado, add a pinch of salt and black pepper, and a squeeze of lime juice.
3. Toast two slices of bread and spread 1 tablespoon of avocado mixture on each slice.
4. Place the bacon on one slice of bread. Add the lettuce and then the tomato.
5. Cut in half on a diagonal.
6. Serve with a dill pickle spear (optional).

Roasted Veggie and Spinach Wrap[49]

Servings: 2; Portion: 1 wrap

Ingredients:

2 large whole wheat tortillas
1 medium zucchini, cut into strips
1 medium yellow squash, sliced
½ cup mushrooms, sliced
1 medium red onion, sliced
1 red bell pepper, cut into strips
2 garlic cloves, sliced
Kosher salt
Black pepper
1 teaspoon smoked paprika

Spinach Spread Ingredients:
1½ cups raw spinach
1 garlic clove, minced
1⁄3 cup plain Greek yogurt
2 teaspoons olive oil
1 tablespoon Parmesan cheese
Kosher salt
Black pepper

How to Make:

1. Preheat oven to 450 degrees.
2. Spread a thin layer of olive oil onto a rimmed baking sheet.
3. Arrange the zucchini, squash, mushrooms, onion, bell pepper, and sliced garlic onto the baking sheet.
4. Sprinkle veggies with kosher salt, black pepper, and smoked paprika.

5. Roast for 30 minutes, or until tender (the roasted veggies can be made ahead of time).

6. While the veggies roast, add the spinach, minced garlic, and yogurt to a food processor until well combined.

7. Add 2 teaspoons of olive oil and Parmesan cheese to the food processor and combine.

8. Season spinach mixture to taste with salt and pepper.

9. Spread the spinach mixture onto each tortilla.

10. Add the roasted vegetables and roll them up.

11. Slice in half and enjoy!

Strawberry Spinach Salad[50]

Ingredients:

2 cups raw spinach
1 cup strawberries, sliced
1 cup raw broccoli florets
¼ cup feta cheese, crumbled
1 tablespoon pecans, chopped
2 tablespoons balsamic vinaigrette dressing

How to Make:

1. Combine spinach, broccoli, feta, pecans, strawberries in a large bowl.
2. Serve by drizzling balsamic vinaigrette over the salad.

Tomato and Turkey Grilled Cheese[51]

<u>Ingredients:</u>

2 slices whole wheat bread
Turkey breast, sliced
1 small tomato, sliced
2 slices Swiss cheese

<u>How to Make:</u>

1. Add the ingredients in this order to build the sandwich: bread, turkey, tomato, cheese, bread.
2. Spray a panini press or nonstick skillet with cooking spray.
3. Add the sandwich and remove once the bread is golden brown on both sides and the cheese is melted.
4. Serve with 1 serving of veggie chips.

Cranberry Orange Kale Salad[52]

Servings: 3; Portion: 1 bowl

Ingredients:

2 tablespoons olive oil
1 cup dried cranberries
2 tablespoons red wine vinegar
2 teaspoons honey
Juice and zest of half a lemon
¼ teaspoon kosher salt
¼ teaspoon black pepper
1 bunch kale, sliced thin
¼ cup sliced almonds
1 can mandarin oranges, drained

How to Make:

1. In a large bowl, toss the kale with olive oil and salt.
2. Massage kale with your fingers for 1 minute until tender.
3. Add cranberries, red wine vinegar, honey, lemon juice, lemon zest, and stir to combine.
4. Top with the oranges and season with black pepper.

Tuna Salad Croissanwich

Servings: 2; Portion: 1 croissanwich and ½ cup of seedless grapes

Ingredients:

2 cans tuna in water
1 boiled egg, chopped
2 tablespoons celery, minced
1 teaspoon parsley, minced
⅓ cup olive oil mayonnaise
1 tablespoon whole grain mustard
2 tablespoons sweet pickle relish
Black pepper
Kosher salt
2 large croissants, halved lengthwise
2 green leaf lettuce leaves
1 tomato, sliced

How to Make:

1. Add the tuna to a bowl and break it up with a fork.
2. Stir in the celery, parsley, and egg.
3. Add the mayonnaise, mustard, and pickle relish.
4. Season to taste with salt and pepper.
5. Stir to combine.
6. Assemble the sandwiches by arranging the ingredients in this order: croissant half, lettuce leaf, tomato slices, tuna salad, croissant half.
7. Serve with seedless grapes.

Thai Noodle Salad[53]

Servings: 4; Portion: 1 bowl

Ingredients:

1 package soba noodles
2 teaspoons of sesame oil
⅓ cup light soy sauce
3 tablespoons olive oil
1 fresh squeezed lime and the zest from 1 lime
⅓ cup rice wine vinegar
2 tablespoons brown sugar
½ cup cilantro, chopped
2 cloves garlic, minced
¼ cup unsalted peanuts, chopped
2 teaspoons red pepper flakes
½ cup shredded carrots
½ cup thinly sliced cabbage

How to Make:

1. Boil noodles according to package directions. Drain and rinse the noodles with cold water and set aside.
2. Add the sesame oil, rice vinegar, soy sauce, lime juice, lime zest, brown sugar, garlic, and red pepper flakes to a bowl and stir until sugar dissolves.
3. Toss in the carrots, cabbage, peanuts, and cilantro.
4. Add the noodles to the dressing mixture.
5. Cover and refrigerate to chill.
6. Toss the salad before serving.

Skinny Shrimp Po' Boy[54]

<u>Ingredients:</u>

⅛ teaspoon kosher salt
8 medium shrimp, peeled and deveined
1 wheat hoagie roll
¼ teaspoon freshly ground black pepper
¼ teaspoon smoked paprika
¼ teaspoon garlic powder
2 teaspoons extra-virgin olive oil
1 small tomato, sliced
½ cup shredded lettuce
1 teaspoon olive oil mayonnaise
1 teaspoon ketchup
½ teaspoon hot sauce

<u>How to Make:</u>

1. Heat a nonstick skillet to medium-high heat with the olive oil.

2. Season the shrimp with the salt, pepper, garlic powder, and smoked paprika.

3. Add shrimp to the skillet and cook until they turn pink.

4. Remove from the skillet.

5. Mix the mayonnaise, ketchup, and hot sauce and then smear on both sides of the hoagie roll.

6. Add the shrimp and then dress the po' boy by adding the lettuce and tomato.

7. Serve with a dill pickle spear.

21 Dinners

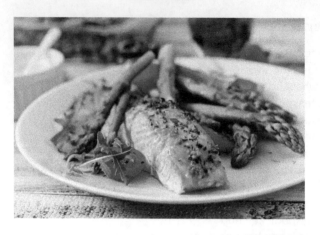

Pack your bags! We will be traveling to exotic dinner destinations for a few weeks. Get ready to savor the flavors. Clean eating is NOT boring and bland!

General Principle: The simpler recipes are ideal for your fast-paced weekday evenings. Save the more involved recipes for the weekend when you can spend a little more time in the kitchen.

All recipes are single serving unless noted otherwise.

Weekday Recipes

Orange Beef and Veggies[55]

Servings: 4; Portion: 1 bowl

Ingredients:

1 cup uncooked brown rice
1½ pounds beef top sirloin, thinly sliced
3 tablespoons light brown sugar
⅓ cup rice wine vinegar
2 large oranges, squeezed
2 tablespoons orange zest
1 teaspoon kosher salt
¼ cup light soy sauce
1 tablespoon ginger powder
1 teaspoon red pepper flakes
1 cup water
2 tablespoons garlic, minced
1 bag fresh broccoli florets
1 cup fresh baby carrots
½ cup canola oil
½ cup of low sodium beef broth
¼ cup flour
1 teaspoon black pepper

How to Make:

1. Place 1 cup of rice into a rice steamer with 1 cup of water.

2. In a bowl, combine the sugar, soy sauce, orange juice, ginger, garlic, red pepper, and rice wine vinegar and set aside.

3. Slice the sirloin into strips, season with black pepper, and then coat with flour.

4. Add the broccoli, carrots, and beef broth to the wok on medium-high heat.

5. Cover and steam veggies until tender for 5 to 7 minutes.

6. Once tender, place the vegetables in a bowl and set aside.

7. Add canola oil to the wok and add the beef.

8. Brown beef on each side for 2 minutes.

9. Remove the beef from the wok and set aside.

10. Add the juice and spice mixture to the wok and allow it to come to a boil for 3 minutes. Reduce to medium-low heat.

11. Add the beef back to the wok and mix well with the sauce.

12. Add the vegetables and stir.

13. Top with orange zest and allow to simmer for 4 minutes.

14. Serve on a bed of brown rice.

Rosemary Pork Chops, Potato, and Green Bean Sheet Pan Dinner[56]

Servings: 4; Portion: 1 porkchop, ½ cup of potatoes, and ½ cup green beans.

Ingredients:

½ cup olive oil
⅓ cup of red wine vinegar
½ teaspoon sea salt
¼ teaspoon black pepper
4 fresh rosemary sprigs or 2 tablespoons dried rosemary
1 tablespoon light brown sugar
1 tablespoon minced garlic
4 center cut pork chops
Sprinkle of sea salt
Sprinkle of black pepper
6 red potatoes cut into chunks
1 (8-ounce) bag fresh whole green beans

How to Make:

1. Add the olive oil, vinegar, rosemary, garlic, salt, pepper, and brown sugar in a gallon-sized freezer bag.

2. Add the pork chops and potatoes and seal the bag. Coat the pork chops and potatoes with the herb mixture and allow to marinate in the refrigerator for 1 hour if time permits.

3. Line a rimmed baking sheet with foil and spray the foil with cooking spray.

4. Place the pork chops and potatoes on the baking sheet and pour the marinade over them.

5. Nestle the green beans onto the sheet around the pork chops and potatoes.

6. Bake for 30 minutes at 450 degrees until the potatoes are tender and the pork chops are cooked through.

Slow Cooker Pulled Pork Sandwiches with Slaw[57,58]

Servings: 4; Portion: 1 sandwich

<u>Pulled Pork Ingredients:</u>

1 8-ounce can tomato sauce
1 tablespoon apple cider vinegar
2 tablespoons garlic powder
1 tablespoon onion powder
¼ cup honey
1 teaspoon cumin
2 teaspoon chili powder
1 teaspoon cinnamon
1 teaspoon sea salt
1 teaspoon black pepper
1 pork tenderloin with fat removed

<u>Slaw Ingredients:</u>

Zest of ½ lemon
¼ cup lemon juice
¼ cup olive oil
1 tablespoon honey
1 teaspoon sea salt
¼ teaspoon black pepper
1 bag of shredded coleslaw mix
½ cup plain Greek yogurt

How to Make Pulled Pork:

1. Combine the tomato sauce, spices, honey, and wet ingredients together in a bowl to form the sauce.
2. Place the tenderloin in the slow cooker.
3. Pour sauce mixture over the pork tenderloin.
4. Cook on low for 6 to 8 hours.
5. The meat will easily pull apart with a fork once done.

How to Make Slaw:

1. Mix the olive oil, lemon juice, honey, sea salt, black pepper, and yogurt in a bowl to form a dressing.
2. Place the shredded coleslaw mix in a bowl and pour the dressing over it.
3. Add the lemon zest.
4. Toss to combine all the ingredients.
5. Assemble your sandwich by placing the pulled pork and slaw between wheat buns.
6. Serve with an optional mini ear of boiled corn on the cob.

Cook's Note: Leftover coleslaw will be used to make the blackened catfish sandwich lunch recipe.

Skinnier Shrimp Scampi[59]

Servings: 4; Portion: 1 cup of pasta and 8 shrimp.
Serve it with ½ cup steamed broccoli florets.

Ingredients:

4 tablespoons olive oil
½ teaspoon garlic, minced
1 small onion, diced
1 pound large shrimp, peeled and deveined
2 lemons
½ cup white wine
¼ teaspoon red pepper flakes
8 ounces whole wheat angel hair pasta
½ cup Parmesan cheese, grated
1 tablespoon fresh parsley, chopped
½ teaspoon sea salt
½ teaspoon black pepper

How to Make:

1. Boil the angel hair until al dente, drain, and set it aside.

2. In a large nonstick skillet, sauté onion and garlic in the olive oil.

3. Add the shrimp and cook for 3 minutes until they start to change color.

4. Stir in the juice from the lemons, white wine, red pepper flakes, salt, and pepper.

5. Reduce the heat to low and add the pasta.

6. Mix well and top with Parmesan and fresh parsley.

Cook's Note: Leftover shrimp will be used to make the Shrimp Salad lunch recipe.

Quinoa Bowl with Veggies and Sautéed Chicken[60]

Servings: 2; Portion: 1 bowl

Ingredients:

2 sliced baked or grilled boneless skinless chicken breast
1 cup quinoa cooked in low sodium chicken broth
1 cup fresh broccoli florets
1 cup zucchini, diced
1 red pepper, sliced
1 teaspoon garlic powder
1 teaspoon dried oregano
1 teaspoon kosher salt
1 teaspoon black pepper
½ cup olive oil

How to Make:

1. Coat a baking sheet with olive oil.
2. Place the zucchini, broccoli, and red bell pepper on the baking sheet.
3. Season with the garlic powder, salt, and pepper and bake until tender (about 35 minutes).
4. Cook the quinoa according to the package instructions in low sodium chicken broth.
5. Add the ingredients to a bowl in this order: cooked quinoa, sliced chicken, steamed broccoli sautéed red peppers, diced zucchini.
6. Garnish each bowl with a fresh lemon wedge, a drizzle of olive oil, and a pinch of salt and pepper to taste.

Chicken and Veggie Fried Cauliflower[61]

Servings: 2; Portion: 1½ cup

<u>Ingredients:</u>

1½ tablespoons canola oil
3 boneless skinless chicken breasts cut into pieces
1 cup kale, chopped
1 cup broccoli florets
½ cup carrots, sliced thin
3 cups of raw cauliflower, grated (use a cheese grater or food processor)
2 large eggs, beaten
3 tablespoons light soy sauce
1 tablespoon white rice wine vinegar
¼ cup low sodium chicken broth
1 tablespoon sriracha
1 teaspoon garlic, minced

<u>How to Make:</u>

1. Coat the bottom of a large nonstick pan with canola oil and place over medium heat.

2. Season the chicken breasts with sea salt and black pepper and sauté in the skillet.

3. Remove chicken from the skillet once cooked and set aside in a bowl.

4. Add the chicken broth, kale, garlic, carrots, and broccoli florets to the skillet and steam them by placing a lid on the skillet. Once softened, transfer the vegetables to the bowl with the chicken.

5. Heat 1 tablespoon of canola oil and spread the 3 cups of cauliflower over the bottom of the pan. Allow the cauliflower to become tender. Use a wooden spoon

to create a part down the center of the pan.

6. Add the beaten eggs to the center of the pan and cook, stirring occasionally, until the eggs are cooked.

7. Add the chicken, vegetables, soy sauce, vinegar, and sriracha to the pan and toss until well combined.

8. Serve in a bowl.

Optional: Garnish with thinly sliced scallions, toasted sesame seeds, and a drizzle of sesame oil.

Garden Pesto Pizza [62]

Servings: 4; Portion: 2 slices

<u>Ingredients:</u>

1 whole wheat pizza crust (store bought)
4 tablespoons basil pesto sauce (store bought)
1 cup low-fat mozzarella cheese
½ cup mushrooms, sliced
2 roma tomatoes, sliced
1 cup fresh spinach
Black pepper
Garlic powder
¼ cup feta cheese
Olive oil

<u>How to Make:</u>

1. Preheat oven to 400 degrees.
2. Spread 3 to 4 tablespoons of basil pesto onto the crust.
3. Add a layer of spinach.
4. Add a layer of mushrooms.
5. Add tomatoes.
6. Season to taste with black pepper and garlic powder.
7. Add the mozzarella and feta cheese.
8. Drizzle with olive oil and bake for 13 to 14 minutes, or until cheese is melted and crust is golden.
9. Serve with a simple salad and a drizzle of balsamic vinaigrette.

Zoodles with Meat Sauce[63]

Servings: 4; Portion: 1 bowl

<u>Meat Sauce Ingredients:</u>

1 pound ground turkey
1 can diced tomatoes, with juice
1 can tomato sauce
1 can tomato paste
1 teaspoon paprika
¼ teaspoon cayenne pepper
¼ teaspoon cumin
1½ teaspoons kosher salt
1 teaspoon Italian seasoning
½ teaspoon freshly ground black pepper
2 garlic cloves, minced
2 bay leaves
1 small onion, finely chopped
2 tablespoons chopped fresh parsley
Zoodle Ingredients:
6 medium to large zucchini
Vegetable spiralizer
Grated Parmesan cheese

<u>How to Make Meat Sauce:</u>

1. Combine the ground turkey, onion, spices, diced tomatoes, and salt in a large pot over medium-high heat.

2. Use a wooden spoon to break up the ground turkey as it browns.

3. Add the tomato sauce, tomato paste, and bay leaves.

4. Cover and simmer over medium-low, stirring occasionally until slightly thickened.

5. Remove the bay leaves and stir in the parsley.

6. How to Make the Zoodles:

7. Use a vegetable spiralizer to cut the zucchini into noodles.

8. Heat a large skillet over medium-high heat with olive oil.

9. Add the zoodles and sauté for 2 minutes.

10. Add a pinch of kosher salt and a pinch pepper.

To Serve:

1. Add the meat sauce to the skillet and gently mix the zoodles with the sauce.

Optional: Add 2 tablespoons of grated Parmesan cheese and serve.

Creole Jamalaya[64]

Servings: 6; Portion: 1 ½ cup

Ingredients:

2 teaspoons canola oil
4 boneless skinless chicken breasts, cut into chunks
¼ teaspoon sea salt
¼ teaspoon freshly ground black pepper
1½ cup smoked turkey sausage, diced
½ cup onion, chopped
½ cup green bell pepper, chopped
½ cup celery, chopped
2 garlic cloves, minced
1½ cups uncooked brown rice
2¾ cups low sodium chicken broth
2 teaspoons paprika
½ teaspoon dried thyme
¼ teaspoon ground red pepper
1 (14.5-ounce) can diced tomatoes, with juice
¼ pound large shrimp, peeled and deveined
¼ cup thinly sliced green onions for garnish, optional
¼ cup chopped fresh parsley for garnish, optional

How to Make Jambalaya:

1. Heat oil in a dutch oven over medium-high heat.
2. Add chicken and sausage, stirring occasionally until lightly browned.
3. Add the onion, bell peppers, celery, and garlic and cook for 3 minutes until the vegetables are tender.
4. Add the diced tomatoes and spices, stirring occasionally for 3 minutes until it simmers.
5. Mix in the brown rice and cook for 1 minute before

adding the chicken stock. Bring to a boil and then lower to a simmer.

6. Cover and cook for 40 minutes until the rice is tender and most of the liquid has been absorbed.

7. Stir in shrimp, cover, and cook 5 minutes or until shrimp turn pink.

Taco Salad[65]

Servings: 4; Portion: 1 bowl

Ingredients:

1 pound ground turkey
1 tablespoon taco seasoning
¼ cup fresh chopped cilantro
Romaine lettuce, chopped
1 cup reduced-fat Mexican blend shredded cheese
1 cup fresh salsa, store bought
1 cup whole wheat tortilla chips, crumbled
1 lime cut into wedges
1 sliced avocado
1 diced tomato
¼ cup chopped cilantro, optional
2 thinly sliced scallions, optional

How to Make:

1. Heat a nonstick pan on medium-high heat, add the ground turkey, and break it up with a wooden spoon. Add the taco seasoning and cook turkey until brown.

2. Assemble the salad ingredients in the following order: lettuce, ground turkey, tomato, cheese, salsa, crumbled tortilla chips, and 2 slices of avocado.

3. Garnish with chopped cilantro scallions and add the juice from 1 lime wedge.

Oven Roasted Orange Chicken[66]

Servings: 4; Portion: 1 leg quarter and ½ cup green beans

Ingredients:

4 chicken leg quarters
¼ cup olive oil
4 cloves of garlic, minced
2 tablespoons brown sugar
2 lemons, 1 juiced and 1 sliced
2 oranges, 1 juiced and 1 sliced
1 tablespoon Italian seasoning
½ teaspoon paprika
1 teaspoon onion powder
¼ teaspoon crushed red pepper flakes
1 medium onion (any kind), thinly sliced
1 teaspoon thyme, dried or freshly chopped
1 tablespoon rosemary, dried or freshly chopped
Kosher salt and freshly ground pepper, to taste

How to Make:

1. In a small bowl, mix olive oil, Italian seasoning, garlic, sugar, lemon juice, orange juice, onion powder, paprika, red pepper flakes, and salt and pepper.
2. Place chicken in a glass baking dish with skin side up and pour the spice mixture over the chicken.
3. Cover with plastic wrap and allow to marinate for 1 hour.
4. Preheat oven to 400 degrees.
5. After 1 hour, place slices of lemon, orange, and onion around and under the chicken.
6. Sprinkle thyme, rosemary, salt, and pepper on top of chicken.

7. Bake uncovered for 45 minutes. Take a spoon to pour the pan juices over the chicken and bake for another 15 minutes, or until the juices run clear when pierced with a fork.

8. Serve with steamed green beans.

Cook's Note: Leftover orange oven roasted chicken will be used to make the Fresh Harvest Salad lunch recipe.

Baked Salmon and Bacon Wrapped Asparagus Bundles[67,68]

Serving: 6; Portion: 1 3-ounce piece of fish and
1 asparagus bundle

Salmon Ingredients:

1 whole salmon fillet
1 large lemon, sliced
¼ cup chopped parsley
1 small red onion, sliced
2 teaspoons olive oil
½ teaspoon sea salt
½ teaspoon black pepper
3 cloves garlic, minced
Olive oil

Asparagus Bundle Ingredients:
1 bunch of asparagus
10 thin cut bacon slices, cut in half
1 tablespoon olive oil
¼ teaspoon garlic powder
½ teaspoon kosher salt
½ teaspoon black pepper

How to Make:

1. Preheat oven to 425 degrees.
2. Cover a baking pan with foil and place salmon on it, skin side down.
3. Combine the olive oil, salt, pepper, garlic, and parsley into a bowl.
4. Spread herb mixture over salmon.
5. Place the lemon and onion slices on the salmon.
6. Bake uncovered for 16 to18 minutes or until flakes with a fork.

How to Make Asparagus Bundles:

1. Heat oven to 425 degrees.
2. Wrap 4 stalks with a piece of bacon and repeat until all the asparagus has been wrapped.
3. Spray a baking sheet with cooking spray and place the wrapped asparagus on it.
4. Spoon the herbed mixture over the asparagus.
5. Bake until asparagus and bacon are cooked, about 15 minutes.

Cook's Note: Leftover salmon will be used to make the Salmon Salad lunch recipe.

Pecan-Crusted Tilapia and Steamed Spinach[69,70]

Servings: 4; Portion: 1 piece of tilapia and 1 cup of spinach

<u>Pecan-Crusted Tilapia Ingredients:</u>

4- to 6-ounce tilapia fillets
2 cups pecans
½ teaspoon kosher salt
¼ teaspoon pepper
¼ teaspoon garlic powder
¼ teaspoon paprika
2 tablespoons lemon juice

<u>Steamed Spinach Ingredients:</u>

1 tablespoon olive oil
1 bag fresh spinach leaves
¼ teaspoon kosher salt
¼ teaspoon black pepper
¼ teaspoon garlic powder
¼ cup low sodium chicken broth

<u>How to Make Pecan-Crusted Tilapia:</u>
1. Heat oven to 350 degrees.
2. Add pecans, lemon juice, and spices to a food processor and finely chop.
3. Place nut mixture in a freezer bag.
4. Add each tilapia fillet to the bag and shake to coat with the nut mixture.
5. Place the pecan-crusted fillets on an oiled baking sheet.
6. Bake uncovered for 20 minutes, or until golden brown.

How to Make Steamed Spinach:

1. Heat the olive oil in a large skillet over medium heat.

2. Add the spinach, chicken broth, salt, pepper, and garlic to the skillet and cover.

3. Allow to cook 5 minutes, stir with a wooden spoon, and cover for another 3 minutes until spinach is wilted.

Chicken Fiesta Tortilla Soup[71]

Servings: 6; Portion: 1 bowl

<u>Ingredients:</u>

3 whole boneless skinless chicken breasts
1 tablespoon olive oil
1 teaspoon cumin
1 teaspoon chili powder
½ teaspoon garlic powder
½ teaspoon salt
1 cup red onion, diced
½ cup red bell pepper, diced
2 cloves garlic, minced
1 can diced fire roasted tomatoes, drained
1 32-ounce container low sodium chicken stock
1 can black beans, drained
Chopped cilantro, optional
Diced avocado, optional

<u>How to Make:</u>

1. Bring 3 cups of water to a boil.
2. Add chicken breasts, cumin, chili pepper, garlic powder, and salt. Boil for 5 minutes and reduce to medium-low heat.
3. Add onions, red pepper, green pepper, and minced garlic and stir.
4. Add diced tomatoes and black beans. Reduce heat to a simmer and simmer for 45 minutes, uncovered.
5. Stir and taste. Add more chili powder and a pinch of salt if needed.
6. Remove from heat.
7. Ladle into a bowl and garnish with tortilla chips, cilantro, and avocado.

Grilled Lamb Kabobs with Spiced Carrots[72,73]

Servings: 4; Portion: 5 meatballs, ¾ cup carrots

<u>Grilled Lamb Kabobs Ingredients:</u>

6 ounces ground lamb
6 ounces ground sirloin
⅓ cup onion, chopped
¼ cup parsley, chopped
1 tablespoon fresh mint, chopped
½ teaspoon cumin
1 teaspoon lemon zest
Kosher salt
Black pepper
¼ teaspoon ground red pepper
Roasted Spiced Carrot Ingredients:
2 tablespoons olive oil
3 cups of carrots, diagonally cut
Black pepper
Kosher salt
¼ teaspoon cumin
¼ cup parsley, chopped
2 teaspoon lemon juice
½ teaspoon cinnamon
½ teaspoon ground ginger
½ teaspoon brown sugar

<u>How to Make Grilled Lamb Kabobs</u>

1. Combine the meat, fresh herbs, and spices into a mixing bowl.
2. Shape the mixture into 12 meatballs.
3. Place 3 meatballs onto each metal skewer.
4. Gently shape each meatball into an oval shape on the skewer.

5. Coat a grill pan with cooking spray and heat to medium-high heat.

6. Place the skewers on the pan and grill for 9 to 10 minutes until done. Turn occasionally.

How to Make Roasted Spiced Carrots:

1. Preheat oven to 425 degrees.

2. Add carrots, olive oil, spices, and a pinch of salt and pepper to a large zip-top freezer bag.

3. Seal the bag and shake vigorously to coat the carrots.

4. Arrange on a baking sheet and bake for 20 minutes or until carrots are tender.

5. Remove from the oven and drizzle with lemon juice, olive oil, and sprinkle with the parsley before serving.

Cook's Note: Leftover kabobs will be used to make the Loaded Greek Pita lunch recipe.

Weekend Recipes

Jerk Pork Chops with Jamaican Peas and Rice[74,75]

Servings: 4; Portion: 1 pork chop and ½ cup of peas and rice

Peas and Rice Ingredients:

1 cup parboiled rice
1 can kidney beans, rinsed and drained
1 can light coconut milk
1½ cups water
2 cloves garlic, chopped
½ teaspoon dried thyme
½ teaspoon kosher salt, to taste
½ teaspoon black pepper
1 teaspoon allspice
Jerk Pork Chop Ingredients:
4 center-cut pork chops
1 can diced pineapples (put the juice and pineapples in separate bowls)
1 teaspoon allspice
1 teaspoon thyme
½ teaspoon cinnamon
¼ teaspoon nutmeg
1 tablespoon light brown sugar
½ teaspoon kosher salt
½ teaspoon black pepper
½ teaspoon ground red pepper

How to Make Peas and Rice:

1. Add coconut milk, beans, garlic, water, and spices to a large pot and bring to a boil.
2. Add rice and boil on high for 2 minutes.

3. Stir and turn heat to low and cook covered until all liquid is absorbed (about 15 to 20 min).

4. Fluff with fork before serving.

How to Make Jerk Pork Chops:

1. Combine the spices and pineapple juice in a bowl.

2. Preheat the oven to 350 degrees.

3. Rinse the pork chops and pat dry with a paper towel.

4. Heal a large cast iron skillet with 1 tablespoon olive oil.

5. Sear the pork chops on each side.

6. Remove from heat and pour jerk marinade over the pork chops.

7. Place the skillet in the oven, turn the pork chops after 10 minutes, and spoon the marinade over them.

8. After 10 more minutes, turn the pork chops again and place a heaping amount of pineapple on each pork chop.

9. Spoon the marinade over them and bake for 5 more minutes.

Stuffed Acorn Squash and Moroccan Cucumber Salad[76,77]

Servings: 4; Portion: 1 acorn squash and 1 cup of salad

Stuffed Acorn Squash Ingredients:

2 acorn squash
2 teaspoons olive oil
½ pound ground chuck
1 small chopped onion
1 pinch cinnamon
1 pinch nutmeg
1 pinch kosher salt
2 teaspoons garlic, minced
¼ cup golden raisins
¼ cup freshly chopped parsley
¾ cup bulgur wheat

Moroccan Cucumber Salad Ingredients:

2 cups cucumbers, chopped
2 cups tomatoes, chopped
2 tablespoons fresh mint, chopped
2 teaspoons onion, finely chopped
2 tablespoons lemon juice
3 tablespoons olive oil
Sea salt
Pepper

How to Make Stuffed Acorn Squash:

1. Preheat the oven to 400 degrees.
2. Cut the acorn squash in half and remove the seeds with a spoon.
3. Place the squash in a casserole dish (flesh side down) and bake for 40 minutes.

4. While the squash is cooking, brown the ground beef in a pot and add a pinch of cinnamon, salt, and nutmeg to it.

5. Transfer the meat to a bowl and reserve the pot of liquid.

6. Add the onion and garlic to the liquid and cook for 4 minutes.

7. To the pot, add 1 teaspoon of salt, the bulgur, and 2 cups of water and bring to a boil.

8. Reduce to medium heat, cover with a lid, and cook for 15 minutes.

9. Remove from the heat and let the bulgur sit for 5 minutes.

10. Add the ground beef, raisins, and parsley to the bulgur and combine all the ingredients.

11. Scrape out the center of the cooked squash and add it to the beef and bulgur mixture.

12. Divide the mixture evenly in the squash halves.

13. Allow the stuffed squash to bake for 12 minutes until the tops are browned.

How to Make Moroccan Cucumber Salad:

1. Peel the cucumber and remove the seeds before chopping.

2. Remove the seeds from the tomatoes and chop into small pieces.

3. Chop the fresh onion and mint.

4. In a bowl, combine the cucumber, tomato, onion, mint, lemon juice, and olive oil.

5. Add salt and pepper to taste.

6. For more intense flavor, place the salad in the

refrigerator for an hour before serving.

Cook's Note: Leftover Moroccan Cucumber Salad is used to make the Moroccan Quinoa Salad lunch recipe.

Hawaiian Steaks and Baked Sweet Potatoes[78]

Servings: 2; Portion: 1 steak and ½ baked sweet potato

Ingredients:

2 thick cut steaks (rib eye, New York strip, or sirloin)
1 cup low sodium soy sauce
2 garlic cloves, minced
½ cup light brown sugar
6 ounces pineapple juice
⅓ cup apple cider vinegar
2 teaspoons fresh ginger, minced

How to Make:

1. Add the pineapple juice, soy sauce, garlic, brown sugar, and apple cider vinegar to a small pot.
2. Bring to a boil and simmer over low heat for 3 minutes.
3. Remove from heat and pour the marinade into a shallow glass dish and set aside to cool.
4. Once cooled, add the steaks to the dish.
5. Cover with plastic wrap and put in the refrigerator for 1 hour (this step could be completed the day before).
6. After 1 hour, remove from refrigerator and bring steaks to room temperature for 25 minutes.
7. Heat grill or grill pan and grill steaks for 5 minutes.
8. Flip steaks and grill for another 5 minutes or to an internal temperature of 140 degrees for medium.
9. Remove steaks from grill and cover with foil to let them rest for 5 minutes.
10. Serve with a baked sweet potato.

Southern Pot Roast and Mashed Cauliflower[79,80]

Servings: 2; Portion: 2 to 3 slices of pot roast and
¾ cup cauliflower

Pot Roast Ingredients:

1 3-pound boneless round roast
Kosher salt
Black pepper
¼ cup canola oil
2 yellow onions, peeled and quartered
4 cloves garlic, smashed
1 tablespoon tomato paste
1 cup red wine
2 cups beef stock
2 fresh thyme sprigs
2 bay leaves

Mashed Cauliflower Ingredients:

1 medium head of cauliflower
1 tablespoon cream cheese, softened
¼ cup Parmesan cheese, grated
½ teaspoon garlic, minced
½ teaspoon kosher salt
¼ teaspoon black pepper
1 tablespoon olive oil

How to Make Pot Roast:

1. Preheat the oven to 350 degrees.
2. Season the roast on all sides with salt and pepper.
3. Heat canola oil over medium-high heat in a Dutch-oven-style pot and sear the roast on all sides.

4. Add the onions, garlic, tomato paste, wine, beef stock, thyme, and bay leaves. Bring the liquid to a simmer. Cover and place in the oven.

5. Bake roast for 3 hours.

6. Transfer the roast to a cutting board and allow to rest for 20 minutes before slicing.

7. Skim any fat off the braising liquid.

8. Slice the roast and place on a serving platter.

9. Pour the braising liquid over it.

How to Make Mashed Cauliflower:

1. Rinse and cut cauliflower into small pieces.

2. Add to a pot of boiling water and cook for 6 to 8 minutes.

3. Drain well and dry cooked cauliflower very well between several layers of paper towels.

4. Add hot cooked cauliflower, cream cheese, Parmesan cheese, garlic, salt, pepper, and olive oil to a large bowl.

5. Purée in the bowl with an immersion blender or in a food processor until smooth.

Peruvian Whole Chicken with Green Sauce[81]

Servings: 4; Portion: 2 to 3 slices of chicken breast or 2 whole chicken pieces and ¼ cup of green sauce.

<u>Peruvian Chicken Ingredients:</u>

1 4-pound whole chicken
3 garlic cloves, chopped
1 tablespoon ground cumin
1 tablespoon olive oil
1 tablespoon paprika
½ teaspoon freshly ground black pepper
½ teaspoon dried oregano
1 ½ teaspoons kosher salt, divided
2 lemons

<u>Green Sauce Ingredients:</u>

1 cup fresh cilantro leaves with stems
2 medium jalapeños, chopped
1 garlic clove, chopped
1 tablespoon olive oil
2½ teaspoons lime juice
¼ teaspoon kosher salt
½ cup plain Greek yogurt

<u>How to Make Peruvian Chicken:</u>

1. Preheat the oven to 400 degrees.
2. Mix garlic, cumin, olive oil, paprika, pepper, oregano, ½ teaspoon of salt, and the zest from 1 lemon in a medium bowl.
3. Cut the zested lemon into quarters and set aside.
4. Squeeze juice from the second lemon into the spice mixture.

5. Rinse the chicken and place it breast side down, use a pair of kitchen shears to cut along both sides of backbone to remove it, turn chicken breast side up, and then press down on the breastbone with the palm of your hand until you hear it crack. Now the chicken will lay flat.

6. Pat chicken dry with paper towels and rub the chicken with the leftover lemon rinds.

7. Carefully loosen skin from both breasts and thighs and use your fingers to spread 2 tablespoons of the spice mixture under the skin.

8. Season chicken all over with the remaining teaspoon of salt.

9. Lay the chicken flat with the skin side up in a roasting pan lined with foil.

10. Roast chicken for 25 minutes, then brush on the remaining spice mixture.

11. Continue to roast and use a spoon to pour the pan juices and spices over the chicken every 20 minutes.

12. Repeat this process until the juices run clear when you pierce the thigh with a fork or the temperature of the thickest part of the thigh reaches 165 degrees (estimated to take 60 minutes for total cooking time).

13. Transfer chicken to a serving platter and allow to rest 15 minutes. Be sure to save the pan juices.

How to Make the Green Sauce:

1. Purée cilantro, jalapeños, garlic, olive oil, lime juice, and salt in a blender or food processor.

2. Add Greek yogurt and purée until well combined.

3. Transfer to a small bowl, cover, and refrigerate until ready to use.

Serve Peruvian chicken and green sauce with a lettuce, tomato, and cucumber salad.

Cook's Note: Leftover Peruvian chicken will be used to make the Peruvian Chicken Salad lunch recipe.

Blackened Catfish with Collard Greens[82,83]

Servings: 4, Portion: 1 catfish fillet and 1 cup of collard greens

Blackened Catfish Ingredients:

4 farm-raised catfish fillets
2 tablespoons paprika
1 tablespoon dried oregano
½ teaspoon kosher salt
½ teaspoon black pepper
¼ teaspoon ground red pepper
2 teaspoons olive oil

Collard Green Ingredients:

1 bag fresh collard greens, chopped
2 fully cooked, smoked turkey wings
½ onion, diced
3 garlic cloves, diced
3 cups of chicken broth
½ teaspoon red pepper flakes
1 tablespoon olive oil
1 cup water

How to Make Blackened Catfish:

1. Add the spices to a small bowl and stir to combine.
2. Season both sides of the fish with the spice mixture.
3. Heat olive oil in a large cast iron skillet over medium-high heat.
4. Add fish and cook for 6 minutes on each side or until fish flakes easily with a fork.

How to Make Southern Style Collard Greens:

1. In a large pot, sauté onions and garlic in olive oil until tender.
2. Add the water, chicken broth, red pepper flakes, and turkey legs and bring to a boil.
3. Reduce to medium heat and simmer for 25 minutes.
4. Add the collard greens and cook until tender for 45 to 60 minutes.

Cook's Note: Leftover catfish fish will be used for the blackened catfish sandwich lunch recipe.

Snack Ideas[84-88]

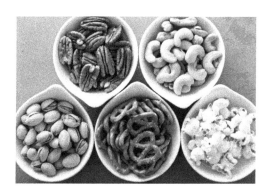

- 1 piece of string cheese and 5 strawberries

- ½ cup guacamole and 10 wheat tortilla chips

- 1 cup fresh melon chunks

- ½ banana with 1 piece of dark chocolate

- 1 green apple sliced in rings with almond butter and dark chocolate chips on top

- fresh baby carrots, cherry tomatoes, and celery with 2 tablespoons low-fat ranch

- ½ cup plain Greek yogurt with ¼ cup fresh blueberries topped with granola

- ½ sliced cucumber and ½ sliced red bell pepper with 3 tablespoons of hummus

- 1 small Gala apple with 1 tablespoon almond butter

- 1 medium pear

- 10 wheat tortilla chips with ½ cup salsa

- 1 Babybel cheese wheel and ½ cup of grapes

- 1 serving Boom Chick Pop popcorn

- 1 serving Boom Chick Puffs cheese puffs

- 1 handful sweet potato chips

- 1 plain rice cake topped with low-fat cream cheese, sliced tomato, and black pepper

- 1 white cheddar rice cake topped with low-fat cream cheese and 1 thin slice of turkey

- 1 plain rice cake topped with part-skim ricotta cheese, fresh blueberries, and a drizzle of honey

- 1 handful of almonds

- 1 wedge of Laughing Cow cheese and 5 whole grain crackers

- 1 fruit and nut granola bar

- 1 cup of mixed fresh fruit

- 1 cup fresh cherries

- 2 granola cracker squares topped with hazelnut spread and a strawberry slice

- 1 handful of trail mix

- 1 handful of walnuts

- 1 cup watermelon chunks

- 2 sliced celery stalks with 2 tablespoons black bean dip

- 1 slice of turkey rolled up inside 1 slice Swiss cheese

- ½ cup kale chips

- ½ cup apple chips

- Sliced celery stuffed with natural peanut butter and raisins

- 2 jumbo pretzel sticks with homemade dip (dip = Greek yogurt, peanut butter, and honey)

- ¼ cup mixed dried fruit and nuts

Busy Woman's Guide –
Week 1 Clean Shopping List

For week 1 Dr. Jamie has made your clean shopping list and checked it twice.

Fruits

Fresh strawberries

1 can chopped pineapple

1 can sugar free fruit cocktail in water

Bananas

1 small cantaloupe

1 bag frozen mixed berries-strawberries, blueberries, raspberries

2 navel oranges

2 lemons

Veggies

Fresh sliced mushrooms

3 roma tomatoes

1 bag fresh spinach

1 zucchini

1 red bell pepper

1 head cauliflower

Red potatoes

Fresh baby carrots

Frozen broccoli florets

1 bag romaine lettuce

1 container cherry tomatoes

1 bunch fresh kale

Fresh parsley

Fresh rosemary

Fresh or frozen long green beans

1 cucumber

Fresh store bought salsa

1 bag fresh cole slaw mix

Whole grains

Whole grain granola

Whole wheat bread

Whole wheat wraps

Whole wheat tortilla chips

Brown rice

Quinoa

Whole wheat angel hair pasta

Whole wheat pizza crust

Dairy

Cottage cheese

Swiss cheese slices

Eggs

Vanilla Greek yogurt

Grated mozzarella cheese

Crumbled feta cheese

Shredded Parmesan cheese

Proteins

1 pound large shrimp

4 center cut pork chops

Boneless skinless chicken breasts

Beef sirloin, thinly sliced	1 jar basil pesto sauce
1 pork tenderloin	1 container hummus
Other	Light soy sauce
1 jar almond butter	Light brown sugar
1 small bag chia seeds	Kosher salt
Coconut flakes	Low sodium beef broth
Roasted almonds with sea salt	Low sodium chicken broth
Boom Chicka Pop Popcorn	1 can low sodium tomato sauce

NOTES

NOTES

NOTES

Acknowledgments

You made it all the way to the end of the book. That's awesome! I'm so, I'm so, I'm so proud of you (in my Drake voice). Of course, this is the part of the book where I have to give my thank yous. So here goes.

Thank YOU for inviting me into your life. Thank YOU for taking me with you to the grocery store as you shopped for ingredients for your clean meals. Thank YOU for bringing me with you to work, to the office, and to school during your lunch break. Thank YOU for making a place for me at the table as you ate dinner. (I am getting teary eyed as I write this). Thank YOU for trusting me to help you transform your eating habits and ultimately your life.

Throughout this process, you have given me so much more than I could have ever hoped for. You may be thinking that in these pages, I gave something to you. The truth is, you allowed me to use my experiences and training to fulfill my purpose of helping busy women to design the life they have always dreamed about. That is PRICELESS!

So now that your eyes have been opened and your taste buds awakened, I need you to remind your best friend, coworkers, and women in your family that they are NOT too busy to eat clean. Go out into the world and help me to spread this message. And when they respond that they are scared and overwhelmed about eating clean, tell them about this guidebook.

Smooches,
Dr. Jamie

References

1. http://www.cdc.gov/chronicdisease/overview/

2. http://www.heart.org/HEARTORG/HealthyLiving/
    HealthyEating/Nutrition/Trans-Fats_UCM_301120_
    Article.jsp#.WA7CB2xSM2w

3. http://www.heart.org/HEARTORG/HealthyLiv-
    ing/HealthyEating/Nutrition/Saturated-Fats_
    UCM_301110_Article.jsp#.V9KfYZgrI2w

4. https://health.gov/dietaryguidelines/2015/guidelines/
    chapter-1/a-closer-look-inside-healthy-eating-pat-
    terns/#fats

5. http://www.fda.gov/NewsEvents/Newsroom/Pres-
    sAnnouncements/ucm451237.htm

6. https://www.choosemyplate.gov/saturated-unsaturat-
    ed-and-trans-fats

7. http://www.heart.org/HEARTORG/HealthyLiv-
    ing/HealthyEating/Nutrition/Sodium-and-Salt_
    UCM_303290_Article.jsp#.WA7D4WxSM2x

8. https://health.gov/dietaryguidelines/2015/guidelines/
    chapter-1/a-closer-look-inside-healthy-eating-pat-
    terns/#sodium

9. https://www.choosemyplate.gov/snapshot-2015-2020-
    dietary-guidelines-america

10. http://www.precisionnutrition.com/create-the-
    perfect-meal-infographic

11. https://health.gov/dietaryguidelines/2015/guidelines/chapter-2/a-closer-look-at-current-intakes-and-rec-ommended-shifts/#beverages

12. http://www.cookinglight.com/eating-smart/smart-choices/clean-eating

13. http://www.mayoclinic.org/healthy-lifestyle/nutri-tion-and-healthy-eating/expert-blog/clean-eating/bgp-20200665

14. http://www.health.com/nutrition/5-reasons-to-eat-healthier-that-have-nothing-to-do-with-your-weight

15. http://www.webmd.com/diet/a-z/eat-clean-diet

16. What We Eat in America, NHANES 2007-2010 for aver-age sugar intakes by age-sex group.

17. Fung, T., et al. 2001. "Association Between Dietary Patterns and Plasma Markers of Obesity and Cardio-vascular Disease Risk." American Journal of Clinical Nutrition 73: 61–67.

18. Brazil Butt Lift Fat Burning Foods

19. www.betterbodyfoods.com/recipes/garden-egg-scramble/

20. www.eatingbirdfood.com/cantaloupe-breakfast-bowls/

21. www.greatist.com/eat/green-smoothie-recipes

22. www.foodnetwork.com/recipes/food-network-kitch-ens/mixed-berries-and-banana-smoothie-recipe.html

23. www.delish.com/cooking/recipe-ideas/recipes/

a45382/avocado-egg-boats-recipe/

24. www.popsugar.com/fitness/Chia-Pudding-Rec-ipe-34333463

25. www.gimmedelicious.com/2016/07/10/how-to-make-the-best-avocado-toast-with-eggs/

26. www.popsugar.com/fitness/Pitaya-Bowl-Reci-pes-37474150#photo-37474150

27. www.happybeinghealthy.com/tag/peaches-and-cream-overnight-oats/

28. www.allrecipes.com/recipe/87817/broiled-grape-fruit/

29. www.gimmedelicious.com/2014/04/11/healthy-low-fat-whole-wheat-banana-pancakes/

30. www.eatingwell.com/recipes/18097/bread/muffins/

31. www.cookinglight.com/food/recipe-finder/snack-bar-recipes

32. www.redbookmag.com/food-recipes/recipes/a35706/huevos-rancheros-bowl-recipe-rbk0413/

33. www.rachaelsgoodeats.com/peanut-butter-banana-chocolate-chip-protein-waffles/

34. www.whitneybond.com/2016/02/16/turkey-egg-breakfast-skillet-recipe/

35. www.eatingwell.com/recipe/249872/salmon-salad/

36. www.foodiecrush.com/mediterranean-quinoa-salad/

37. www.foodandwine.com/recipes/lemony-shrimp-salad

38. www.cookinglight.com/cooking-101/techniques/cheeseburger-salad

39. www.damndelicious.net/2012/11/07/lightened-up-greek-yogurt-chicken-salad-sandwich/

40. www.foodnetwork.com/recipes/bobby-flay/chopped-apple-salad-with-toasted-walnuts-blue-cheese-and-pomegranate-vinaigrette-recipe.html

41. www.skinnymom.com/recipe-lighter-tartar-sauce/

42. www.epicurious.com/recipes/food/views/greek-salad-pita-sandwiches-240435

43. www.aliinthevalley.com/5-minute-turkey-avocado-and-hummus-wrap/

44. www.dashingdish.com/recipe/10-minute-black-bean-corn-quesadillas

45. www.foodnetwork.com/recipes/rachael-ray/black-bean-and-corn-salad-recipe.html

46. www.minq.com/food/19649/13-ways-to-make-your-favorite-sandwiches-without-using-bread/#page=1

47. www.allrecipes.com/recipe/232211/pesto-pasta-caprese-salad/

48. www.skinnytaste.com/blt-with-avocado/

49. www.food.com/recipe/roasted-or-grilled-vegetable-wraps-173074

50. www.wholefoodsmarket.com/recipe/spinach-and-strawberry-salad

51. www.smartbalance.com/recipes/good-you-grilled-cheese-turkey-tomato

52. www.deliciouslyorganic.net/kale-salad-cranberry-vinaigrette-walnuts/

53. www.allrecipes.com/recipe/83087/oriental-cold-noodle-salad/

54. www.skinnytaste.com/slimmed-down-shrimp-po-boy/

55. www.allrecipes.com/recipe/57966/crispy-orange-beef/

56. www.rachaelraymag.com/recipe/roast-pork-chops-with-green-beans-and-potatoes/

57. www.skinnyms.com/slow-cooker-bbq-pulled-pork/

58. www.pbs.org/food/fresh-tastes/no-mayo-coleslaw/

59. www.skinnymom.com/skinny-scampi/

60. www.foodnetwork.com/recipes/roasted-vegetable-and-chicken-quinoa-bowls-for-two.html

61. www.familyfreshmeals.com/2013/03/cauliflower-fried-rice.html

62. www.allrecipes.com/recipe/228983/fresh-pesto-pizza/

63. www.eatyourselfskinny.com/zucchini-noodles-with-simple-bolognese-sauce-2/

64. www.myrecipes.com/recipe/chicken-shrimp-jambalaya

65. www.tasteofhome.com/recipes/turkey-taco-salad

66. www.allrecipes.com/recipe/167419/orange-herb-roasted-chicken/

67. www.cooks.com/recipe/hs46h4fd/baked-salmon-with-lemon-parsley-sauce.html

68. www.foodnetwork.com/recipes/trisha-yearwood/asparagus-bundles-recipe.html

69. www.nola.com/food/index.ssf/2016/02/pecan-crusted_tilapia_recipe.html

70. www.simplyrecipes.com/recipes/spinach/

71. www.thepioneerwoman.com/cooking/chicken-tortilla-soup/

72. www.cookinglight.com/food/world-cuisine/israeli-recipes/zaatar-roasted-carrots-labne

73. www.cookinglight.com/food/world-cuisine/israeli-recipes/grilled-lamb-kufta-kebabs

74. www.cooklikeajamaican.com/rice-and-peas/

75. www.marthastewart.com/340386/jerk-pineapple-pork-chops

76. www.marthastewart.com/1049761/moroccan-style-stuffed-acorn-squashes

77. www.cookinglight.com/food/world-cuisine/israeli-recipes/chopped-israeli-salad

78. www.bonappetit.com/recipe/hawaiian-rib-eye-steak

79. www.foodnetwork.com/recipes/patrick-and-gina-neely/momma-neelys-pot-roast-recipe.html

80. www.foodnetwork.com/recipes/mock-garlic-mashed-potatoes-recipe.html

81. www.epicurious.com/recipes/food/views/peruvian-style-roast-chicken-with-tangy-green-sauce

82. www.food.com/recipe/blackened-catfish-91450

83. www.skinnyms.com/healthy-collard-greens/

84. http://www.100daysofrealfood.com/2012/07/31/85-snacks-for-kids-and-adults/

85. http://www.cookinglight.com/eating-smart/smart-choices/healthy-snacks

86. http://greatist.com/health/high-protein-snacks-portable

87. http://www.womenshealthmag.com/weight-loss/control-portion-size-for-healthy-weight-loss/slide/10

88. http://www.bodybuilding.com/content/26-best-healthy-snacks.html

About the Author

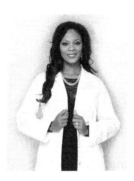

Dr. Jamie J. Hardy, PharmD, BCPS, MS, is a practicing clinical pharmacist, highly sought-after speaker, author, and health correspondent who is passionate about transforming the lives of women all over the globe. Known as The Lifestyle Pharmacist, she helps young women who are busy juggling careers, businesses, and relationships to be fit, fabulous, and fulfilled without prescribed pills. Through her videos, books, and programs, she equips them with the tools necessary to make lasting changes in their lifestyle and design the life of their dreams.

Dr. Jamie obtained her doctorate of pharmacy from Xavier University of Louisiana and her master of science in pharmacy leadership from the University of Florida, and she completed a PGY1 Residency at LSU Health Science Center in New Orleans. She is the founder and chief lifestyle curator of Innovative Wellness LLC, a lifestyle company that provides coaching and live workshops to teach women how to detox, find balance, eat healthier, and effectively manage stress. Her community of followers is affectionately known as The Fab Squad. To name a few of her many accomplishments, Dr. Jamie authored 26 Ways to Eat Clean and Stay Clean, was a featured health and lifestyle contributor for the New Tri-State Defender Newspaper, and was named a Woman to Watch by the Memphis Minority Business Journal.

Along with engaging women through her lifestyle-centric content, Dr. Jamie enjoys gardening, planning events, traveling, exercising, and trying new recipes. She currently resides in Memphis, Tennessee.

To connect, visit her website at:
www.DrJamieHardy.com

CREATING DISTINCTIVE BOOKS
WITH INTENTIONAL RESULTS

We're a collaborative group of creative masterminds
with a mission to produce high-quality books to position
you for monumental success in the marketplace.

Our professional team of writers, editors, designers,
and marketing strategists work closely together to ensure
that every detail of your book is a clear representation
of the message in your writing.

Want to know more?
Write to us at info@publishyourgift.com
or call (888) 949-6228

Discover great books, exclusive offers, and more at
www.PublishYourGift.com

Connect with us on social media

@publishyourgift

CPSIA information can be obtained
at www.ICGtesting.com
Printed in the USA
LVHW01s1333190917
549236LV00002B/2/P